Pre-exam Preparation
for
MEDICINE

Pre-exam Preparation *for* MEDICINE

HN Sarker
MBBS FCPS (Medicine) MRCP (UK) FRCP (Edin)
Associate Professor
Department of Medicine
Sher-e-Bangla Medical College
Barisal, Bangladesh

JAYPEE *The Health Sciences Publishers*

New Delhi | London | Philadelphia | Panama

Jaypee Brothers Medical Publishers (P) Ltd

Headquarters

Jaypee Brothers Medical Publishers (P) Ltd
4838/24, Ansari Road, Daryaganj
New Delhi 110 002, India
Phone: +91-11-43574357
Fax: +91-11-43574314
Email: jaypee@jaypeebrothers.com

Overseas Offices

J.P. Medical Ltd
83 Victoria Street, London
SW1H 0HW (UK)
Phone: +44 20 3170 8910
Fax: +44 (0)20 3008 6180
Email: info@jpmedpub.com

Jaypee Medical Inc
The Bourse
111 South Independence Mall East
Suite 835, Philadelphia, PA 19106, USA
Phone: +1 267-519-9789
Email: jpmed.us@gmail.com

Jaypee Brothers Medical Publishers (P) Ltd
Bhotahity, Kathmandu, Nepal
Phone: +977-9741283608
Email: kathmandu@jaypeebrothers.com

Jaypee-Highlights Medical Publishers Inc
City of Knowledge, Bld. 237, Clayton
Panama City, Panama
Phone: +1 507-301-0496
Fax: +1 507-301-0499
Email: cservice@jphmedical.com

Jaypee Brothers Medical Publishers (P) Ltd
17/1-B Babar Road, Block-B, Shaymali
Mohammadpur, Dhaka-1207
Bangladesh
Mobile: +08801912003485
Email: jaypeedhaka@gmail.com

Website: www.jaypeebrothers.com
Website: www.jaypeedigital.com

Inquiries for bulk sales may be solicited at: jaypee@jaypeebrothers.com

Pre-exam Preparation for Medicine

First Edition: **2015**

ISBN 978-93-5152-549-3

Printed at Rajkamal Electric Press, Plot No. 2, Phase-IV, Kundli, Haryana.

Dedicated to

My parents, wife and children

Preface

Every student must have to pass through the viva table to be a doctor. There are a lot of books and they read much but a few students can produce perfectly because of not formulating as viva. This book is written to help the students to prepare for viva examination within a short time in the form of questions and answers.

My endeavor will be fruitful, if the book helps any student to pass his/her examination successfully.

HN Sarker

Acknowledgments

I am grateful to my students who inspire me to write this book.

I am also grateful to Professor (Dr) Saiyeedur Rahman, Professor and Head, Department of Medicine, SBMC, Barisal, who always appreciate me to all creative works.

I would like to thank my Registrar, Assistant Registrar, IMO, HMO, and Intern doctors who cordially cooperate me to prepare this book.

My special thanks go to Dr Md Siddiqur Rahman, Assistant Professor of Medicine who is always with me to inspire.

I express my thanks to my wife and children for their patience and cooperation.

Contents

CHAPTER 1

Cardiovascular System

Q.1. What are the common presentations of cardiovascular diseases?

Ans. Common presentations are:
- Chest pain
- Breathlessness
- Palpitation
- Edema
- Syncope
- Fatigue
- Hypertension
- Cardiogenic shock.

Q.2. What are the causes of chest pain?

Ans. Causes of chest pain are:
- Central chest pain:
  i. Cardiac chest pain:
    - Myocardial ischemia (angina) and myocardial infarction
    - Pericarditis
    - Mitral valve prolapse.
  ii. Aortic—Aortic dissection.
  iii. Pulmonary/mediastinal—Massive pulmonary embolism and tracheitis.
  iv. Esophageal—Esophagitis.
  v. Musculoskeletal—Osteoarthritis.
  vi. Anxiety/cardiac neurosis.
- Peripheral chest pain:
  i. Lung/pleura:
    - Pneumonia
    - Pneumothorax

  - Malignancy
  - Tuberculosis
  - Pulmonary infarction.

ii. Chest wall disorders:
  - Rib fracture/injury
  - Intercostal muscle injury
  - Costochondritis (Tietze's syndrome)
  - Epidemic myalgia (Bornholm disease).

iii. Psychogenic—Anxiety.

iv. Musculoskeletal:
  - Herpes zoster
  - Herniated intervertebral disk.

Q.3. What is the central chest pain?

Ans. Pain behind the sternum is known as central chest pain.

Q.4. What are the causes of retrosternal chest pain?

Ans. The causes of retrosternal chest pain are:
- Myocardial infarction
- Angina
- Pericarditis
- Aortic dissection
- Esophageal spasm.

Q.5. What are the differences between angina and MI chest pain?

Ans.

Characteristics	Angina	Myocardial infarction
Duration	Short, usually<10 min	Long, usually>20 min
Precipitated	By exercise or emotion	Often spontaneous
Relieved by	Rest, nitrates	Not by rest or nitrates
Sympathetic activity	None	Increased (e.g. sweating)
Nausea or vomiting	Unusual	Common

Q.6. What are the causes of cardiac chest pain?

Ans. The causes of cardiac chest pain are:
- Stable angina
- Unstable angina
- Myocardial infarction
- Pericarditis.

Q.7. How can you differentiate between ischemic cardiac chest pain and nonischemic/noncardiac chest pain?

Ans.

Characteristics	Ischemic cardiac chest pain	Noncardiac chest pain
Site	Central, diffuse	Peripheral, localized
Character	Tight, squeezing, choking	Sharp, stabbing, catching
Radiation	Jaw/neck/shoulder/arm	No radiation/other
Precipitation	By exertion/emotion	By posture, respiration or movement/palpation
Relieving factors	Rest, nitrate	Not relieved by rest, slow or no response to nitrates
Associated features	Breathlessness	Respiratory, GI or locomotors

Q.8. What are the differences between cardiac and esophageal pain?

Ans.

Characteristics	Cardiac pain(angina)	Esophageal pain
Site	Retrosternal; radiates to arm and jaw	Retrosternal or epigastric; may radiate to back
Precipitated	By exertion	This may be worsened by exertion, heavy meal and lying position
Relieved	Rapidly relieved by rest, nitrates	Not rapidly relieved by rest; often relieved by nitrates
Wakes patient from sleep	Rare	Often
Relation to heartburn	No	Sometimes
Duration	Upto10 min	Variable

Q.9. What is angina pectoris?

Ans. Ischemic cardiac chest pain is called angina pectoris.

Q.10. What are the causes of angina?

Ans. Causes of angina are:

- Impaired myocardial oxygen supply
  - Coronary artery disease, e.g. atherosclerosis
  - Coronary artery spasm
  - Congenital coronary artery disease
  - Severe anemia.
- Increased myocardial oxygen demand
  - Left ventricular hypertrophy
    - Hypertension
    - Aortic valve disease
    - Hypertrophic cardiomyopathy
  - Tachyarrhythmias.

Q.11. What are the common causes of angina?

Ans. The common causes of angina are:

- Coronary artery disease
- Aortic stenosis
- Hypertrophic cardiomyopathy.

Q.12. What are the types of angina?

Ans. The types of angina are:

- Stable angina
- Unstable angina
- Prinzmetal's angina
- Nocturnal or decubitus angina.

Q.13. A 35-year-old man who is smoker, hypertensive feels chest pain on walking which radiates to left arm but relieves after standing for a while. What is your diagnosis?

Ans. Stable angina.

Q.14. Describe a typical stable angina.

Ans. A typical stable angina is a retrosternal choking or constricting chest pain, comes on with exertion, is relieved by rest or nitroglycerin, may radiate to jaw, neck or arms (more in left arm).

Q.15. What are the aggravating factors of angina?

Ans. Aggravating factors of angina are:

- Exertion
- Emotional excitement
- Cold weather
- Exercise after meals or heavy meals
- Anemia
- Thyrotoxicosis.

Q.16. What are the relieving factors of angina?

Ans. The relieving factors of angina are:
- Rest
- Glyceryl trinitrate
- Warm-up before exercise.

Q.17. What are the clinical manifestations of coronary heart disease?

Ans. The clinical manifestations of coronary heart disease are:
- Stable angina
- Unstable angina
- Myocardial infarction
- Heart failure
- Arrhythmia
- Sudden death.

Q.18. What is the most common cause of angina?

Ans. The most common cause of angina is coronary atherosclerosis.

Q.19. What is the pathology of stable angina?

Ans. Ischemia due to fixed atheromatous stenosis of one or more coronary arteries, i.e. demand led angina.

Q.20. What are the angina with normal coronary arteries?

Ans. Angina with normal coronary arteries are:
- Prinzmetal's angina (variant angina)
- Syndrome X.

Q.21. What is Prinzmetal's angina?

Ans. Prinzmetal's angina is also known as variant angina, characterized by chest pain at rest that occurs in cycles, due to vasospasm and may be accompanied by spontaneous and transient ST elevation on the ECG.

Q.22. How can you treat Prinzmetal's angina?

Ans. Calcium channel blockers and nitrates.

Q.23. Which antianginal drug is contraindicated in Prinzmetal's angina?

Ans. β-blocker is contraindicated in Prinzmetal's angina.

Q.24. What is cardiac syndrome X?

Ans. Cardiac syndrome X is the constellation of typical angina on effort, objective evidence of myocardial ischemia on stress testing, and angiographically normal coronary arteries.

Q.25. What is the treatment of cardiac syndrome X?

Ans. This is treated with antianginal therapy, usually with β-blocker.

Q.26. What are the risk factors for coronary artery disease?

Ans.
- Major risk factors are:
  - Smoking
  - Hypertension
  - Diabetes mellitus
  - Hypercholesterolemia
  - Sedentary lifestyle.
- Other risk factors:
  - Obesity
  - Homocystinemia
  - Excess alcohol intake.
- Fixed risk factors:
  - Age
  - Male sex
  - Family history.

Q.27. How can you investigate this patient?

Ans.
- **Resting ECG:**
  - The ECG is often normal, even in patients with severe coronary artery disease. The most convincing ECG evidence of myocardial ischemia is ST segment depression with or without T-wave inversion.
- **Exercise ECG:**
  - An exercise tolerance test (ETT) is usually performed using a standard treadmill while monitoring the patient's ECG, BP, and general condition.
  - Planar or down-sloping ST segment depression of ≥ 1 mm is indicative of ischemia.
  - Up-sloping ST depression is less specific and often occurs in normal individuals.
- **Other forms of stress testing**:
  - Myocardial perfusion scanning.
  - Stress echocardiography.
- **Coronary arteriography**:
  - This provides detailed anatomical information about the extent and nature of coronary artery disease.
- **Others**:
  - RBS and lipid profile.

Q.28. How can you manage this patient?

Ans.
- **General measures**:
  - Lifestyle advice—Advice to patients with stable angina.
  - Do not smoke.
  - Aim for ideal body weight.
  - Take regular exercise (exercise upto, but not beyond, the point of chest discomfort is beneficial and may promote collateral vessels).
  - Avoid severe unaccustomed exertion and vigorous exercise after a heavy meal or in very cold weather.
  - Take sublingual nitrate before undertaking exertion that may induce angina.
  - Control of risk factors—Such as smoking, hypertension, and hyperlipidemia.
- **Drug therapy**:

1. Antiplatelet therapy
   - Low-dose (75 mg) aspirin
   - Clopidogrel (75 mg daily), if aspirin causes troublesome dyspepsia or other side effects.
2. Antianginal drug treatment
   - Five groups of drugs are used to help relieve or prevent the symptoms of angina:
     a. Nitrates, e.g. isosorbide dinitrate.
     b. β-blockers, e.g. slow-release metoprolol 50–200 mg daily and bisoprolol 5–15 mg daily.
     c. Calcium antagonists, e.g. verapamil and diltiazem.
     d. Potassium channel activators, e.g. nicorandil.
     e. An **If** channel antagonist.

- **Invasive therapy**:
  - Percutaneous coronary intervention (PCI)
  - Coronary artery bypass grafting (CABG).

Q.29. What is the most common side effect of nitrate?

Ans. Headache is the most common side effect of nitrate.

Q.30. How can you treat it?

Ans. We can treat it by using slow release preparation of nitrate and paracetamol may help.

Q.31. What are the contraindications of β-blocker?

Ans. Bronchial asthma, COPD, advanced heart block, peripheral vascular disease, and NYHA class III and IV heart failure.

Q.32. Do you know NYHA classification?

Ans. New York Heart Association classification of heart failure symptom severity.

Class I — No limitations. Ordinary physical activity does not cause undue fatigue, dyspnea or palpitation (asymptomatic left ventricular dysfunction).

Class II — Slight limitation of physical activity. Such patients are comfortable at rest. Ordinary physical activity results in fatigue, palpitation, and dyspnea or angina pectoris (symptomatically 'mild' heart failure).

Class III — Marked limitation of physical activity. Less than ordinary physical activity will lead to symptoms (symptomatically 'moderate' heart failure).

Class IV — Symptoms of congestive heart failure are present, even at rest. With any physical activity increased discomfort is experienced (symptomatically 'severe' heart failure).

Q.33. What are the common side effects of calcium channel blocker?

Ans. The common side effects of calcium channel blocker are:

- Constipation
- Fluid retention (edema)
- Calcium channel antagonists reduce myocardial contractility and can aggravate or precipitate heart failure.

Q.34. How many patients taking calcium channel blocker develop edema?

Ans. About 50% of patient develops edema, more with dihydropyridine than nondihydropyridine.

Q.35. What is tri-vessel disease?

Ans. Tri-vessel disease is atherosclerosis disease involving left anterior descending (LAD) artery, circumflex (CX) and right coronary arteries.

Q.36. What is ACS? Why both of them known as collectively?

Ans. ACS means acute coronary syndrome. Acute coronary syndrome is a term that encompasses both unstable angina and MI (STEMI and NSTEMI).

These two are considered collectively as initial emergency management is same done by using ACS triage therapy. It is also a dynamic process, i.e. unstable angina if not treated appropriately in time, may progress to MI.

Q.37. What is unstable angina?

Ans. Unstable angina is characterized by new-onset or rapidly worsening angina (crescendo angina), angina on minimal exertion or angina at rest in the absence of myocardial damage.

Q.38. What is the pathology of unstable angina?

Ans. Ischemia caused by dynamic obstruction of a coronary artery due to plaque rupture or erosion with superimposed thrombosis (supply-led angina).

Q.39. How can you manage unstable angina?

Ans. To manage unstable angina:

- Patient should be hospitalized
- Bed rest
- Aspirin—300 mg stat, then 75 mg daily
- Clopidogrel—300 mg stat, then 75 mg daily
- β-blocker—
    - Atenolol—50–100 mg daily
    - Metoprolol— 50–100 mg 12 hourly
- Subcutaneous low molecular weight heparin (enoxaparin 1mg/kg 12 hourly).

If pain persists or recurs

- Intravenous nitrates.

If medical treatment fails

- PCI
- CABG.

Q.40. A 50-year-male smoker develops sudden severe chest pain which radiates to neck. He vomited several times and now he is sweating. What is your diagnosis?

Ans. Acute myocardial infarction.

Q.41. What is myocardial infarction (MI)?

Ans. Acute ischemic necrosis of an area of myocardium is called myocardial infarction.

Q.42. What is the pathology of MI?

Ans. Myocardial necrosis caused by acute occlusion of a coronary artery due to plaque rupture or erosion with superimposed thrombosis.

Q.43. How may a patient with MI present to you?

Ans.

- Prolonged cardiac pain >30 minutes: Chest, throat, arms, and epigastrium or back.
- Breathlessness.
- Collapse/syncope.

- Anxiety and fear of impending death.
- Nausea and vomiting.

Q.44. Please tell WHO diagnostic criteria of MI.

Ans. According to the WHO criteria as revised in 2000, a cardiac troponin rise accompanied by either typical symptoms, pathological Q-waves, and ST elevation or depression or coronary intervention are diagnostic of MI.

Q.45. What is silent MI?

Ans. Painless MI is called silent MI.

Q.46. Who are more prone to develop silent MI?

Ans. Older patients or those with diabetes mellitus.

Q.47. What is the cause of silent MI?

Ans. Autonomic neuropathy.

Q.48. How will you investigate this patient?

Ans. Investigate the patient by:

- ECG
- Cardiac markers
- Blood tests—CBC, ESR, CRP, blood sugar, and lipid profile
- X-ray chest PA view
- Echocardiography.

Q.49. What are the ECG findings in MI?

Ans. The ECG findings in MI are:

- ST segment elevation with convexity upward > 1mm in limb leads, and >2 mm in chest leads
- Diminution of R-wave
- Pathological Q-wave
- Symmetrical T-wave inversion.

Q.50. In which leads do you expect changes of inferior MI?

Ans. Lead II, III, and AVF.

Q.51. In which leads do you expect changes of anterior MI?

Ans. V_{1-6}, I, and AVL.

Q.52. In which leads do the ECG changes occur in acute anteroseptal MI?

Ans. V_{1-4}.

Q.53. In which leads do the ECG changes occur in acute anterolateral MI?

Ans. V_{4-6}.

Q.54. What are the criteria of pathological Q-wave?

Ans. The criteria of pathological Q-wave are:
- Q-wave height >3 mm
- Q-wave wide >1 mm
- Q-wave is more than 25% of the succeeding R-wave.

Q.55. What are the cardiac markers?

Ans. Commonly used cardiac markers are (according to time of appearance):
- Troponin T/I
- CK-MB
- AST
- LDH.

Q.56. How can you manage this patient?

Ans. Early/immediate medical management—first 12 hours:
- Admit the patient in CCU.
- Assess clinically.
- Attach ECG monitor.
- Oxygen inhalation—High concentration/nasal cannula 4–6 L/minute.
- Intravenous access + blood for markers (plus FBC, biochemistry, lipids, and glucose).
- Intravenous opiate, e.g. morphine (or diamorphine) 5–10 mg + antiemetic, e.g. metoclopramide 10 mg, titrated by giving repeated small aliquots until the patient is comfortable.

Antiplatelet therapy:
- Aspirin—The first tablet (300 mg) should be given orally within the first 12 hours and therapy should be continued indefinitely if there are no side effects.
- In combination with aspirin, the early (within 12 hours) use of clopidogrel 600 mg, followed by 150 mg daily for 1 week and 75 mg daily thereafter.
- Anticoagulants—Low molecular weight heparin (subcutaneous enoxaparin 1 mg/kg 12-hourly) should be continued for 8 days or until discharge from hospital or coronary revascularization.

Antianginal therapy:
- Sublingual glyceryl trinitrate 0.3–1 mg. Repeat if necessary.
- β-blocker (if no contraindication) for ongoing chest pain, hypertension, and tachycardia.

Reperfusion therapy:
- If primary PCI available, give GP IIb/IIIa inhibitor then PCI.
- Alternatively give thrombolysis.

Q.57. What drugs are used to relief pain in MI?
Ans. Opiate, e.g. morphine or diamorphine.

Q.58. What are the contraindications of morphine?
Ans. The contraindications of morphine are bronchial asthma, COPD, respiratory depression, and profound hypotension.

Q.59. What are the thrombolytic agents?
Ans. Alteplase, streptokinase, tenecteplase, and reteplase.

Q.60. Which is commonly used in our country?
Ans. Streptokinase.

Q.61. What are the indications of thrombolytic therapy?
Ans. Patients with MI presenting within 12 hours of the onset of symptoms and PCI is unavailable.
ECG shows—
1. New onset left bundle branch block or
2. Characteristic ST segment elevation > 1 mm in the limb leads or 2 mm in the chest leads.

Q.62. What are the contraindications of thrombolytic therapy?
Ans. The contraindications of thrombolytic therapy are:
- Active internal bleeding.
- Previous subarachnoid or intracerebral hemorrhage.
- Uncontrolled hypertension.
- Recent surgery (within 1 month).
- Recent trauma (including traumatic resuscitation).
- High probability of active peptic ulcer.
- Pregnancy.

Q.63. How is streptokinase given?
Ans. 1.5 million units mixed in 100 mL of normal saline infuse intravenously over 1 hour.

Q.64. What are the side effects/complications of streptokinase?
Ans. The side effects/complications of streptokinase are:
- Bleeding such as stroke.
- Transient hypotension.

Q.65. What are the immediate complications of MI?
Ans. The immediate complications of MI are:

- Arrhythmia
- Ischemia
- Cardiogenic shock.

Q.66. What are the complications of MI?

Ans. i. Early complications are:
- Arrhythmia—All types of arrhythmia
- Ischemia
- Cardiogenic shock
- Pericarditis
- Thromboembolism

ii. Mechanical complications are:
- Rupture of chorda tendinae or papillary muscle damage leading to MR
- Rupture of interventricular septum leading to VSD.

iii. Late complications are:
- Ventricular aneurysm
- Dressler's syndrome (pleurisy, pericarditis, and pyrexia-3P)
- Shoulder hand syndrome.

Q.67. What is the late management of MI?

Ans.
1. Risk stratification and further investigation.
2. Lifestyle modification—
   - Cessation of smoking
   - Regular exercise
   - Diet (weight control and lipid-lowering).
3. Secondary prevention drug therapy—
   - Antiplatelet therapy (aspirin and/or clopidogrel)
   - β-blocker
   - ACE inhibitor/ARB
   - Statin.
4. Additional therapy for control of diabetes and hypertension.
5. Aldosterone receptor antagonist.
6. Rehabilitation devices—Implantable cardiac defibrillator for high-risk patients.

Q.68. What are the roles of ACE inhibitor in MI?

Ans. ACE inhibitor can counteract ventricular remodeling and thus—

a. Prevent the onset of heart failure
b. Improve survival
c. Reduce recurrent MI
d. Avoid rehospitalization.

Q.69. What are the roles of β-blocker in MI?

Ans. β-blocker can—

a. Relieve pain
b. Reduce arrhythmias
c. Reduce blood pressure
d. Improve short-term mortality in patients who present within 12 hours of the onset of symptoms.

Q.70. What are the causes of sudden severe chest pain?

Ans. The causes of sudden severe chest pain are:

- Dissecting aortic aneurysm
- Tension pneumothorax
- Pulmonary embolism.

Q.71. What is dyspnea?

Ans. Dyspnea (breathlessness) is a subjective awareness of increased drive to breathe.

Q.72. What are the causes of acute dyspnea?

Ans. i. Cardiac causes:
  - Acute pulmonary edema
  - Myocardial ischemia.

ii. Respiratory causes:
  - Acute severe asthma
  - Acute exacerbation of chronic obstructive pulmonary disease
  - Pneumothorax
  - Pneumonia
  - Pulmonary embolism
  - Acute respiratory distress syndrome
  - Laryngeal edema (e.g. anaphylaxis).

iii. Others:
  Psychogenic hyperventilation, metabolic acidosis (e.g. diabetic ketoacidosis, lactic acidosis, uremia, overdose of salicylates, and ethylene glycol poisoning).

Q.73. What are the causes of chronic dyspnea or dyspnea on exertion?

Ans. i. Cardiac causes:
  - Chronic congestive cardiac failure.
  - Chronic pulmonary thromboembolism.

ii. Respiratory causes:
  - Chronic obstructive pulmonary disease.
  - Chronic asthma.
  - Bronchial carcinoma.

- Interstitial lung diseases: Sarcoidosis, fibrosing alveolitis.
- Large pleural effusion(s).

iii. Others:
- Severe anemia.
- Obesity.

Q.74. What are the causes of acute pulmonary edema or acute left heart failure?

Ans. Acute left heart failure due to:

1. Myocardial infarction
2. Systemic hypertension
3. Acute mitral regurgitation due to rupture of chordae tendineae
4. Myocarditis.

Acute on chronic heart failure:

1. Mitral stenosis
2. Aortic stenosis.

Q.75. A 60-year-old man wakes up with shortness of breath at midnight and rushes toward the window. He feels better after several minutes after coughing up small frothy sputum. What is your diagnosis?

Ans. Paroxysmal nocturnal dyspnea due to left ventricular failure.

Q.76. What are the clinical features of acute pulmonary edema?

Ans. The clinical features of acute pulmonary edema are:

- Dyspnea at rest
- Paroxysmal nocturnal dyspnea (PND)
- Orthopnea
- Perspiration
- Cyanosis
- Pulsus alternans
- Gallop rhythm
- Bilateral basal crepitation
- Features of underlying cause.

Q.77. What is orthopnea?

Ans. Orthopnea is dyspnea on lying flat.

Q.78. What are the characteristics of sputum in acute pulmonary edema?

Ans. Frothy sputum may be tingned with blood.

Q.79. How can you manage acute pulmonary edema?

Ans.
1. Urgent hospitalization.
2. Sit the patient up in order to reduce pulmonary congestion.
3. Give oxygen (high-flow, and/or high-concentration).
4. Administer nitrates, such as IV glyceryl trinitrate 10–200 µg/minute or buccal glyceryl trinitrate 2–5 mg, titrated upwards every 10 minute, until clinical improvement occurs or systolic BP falls to < 110 mmHg.
5. Administer a loop diuretic such as furosemide 40–80 mg IV.
6. Intravenous opiates may be cautiously used when patients are in extremes. They reduce sympathetically mediated peripheral vasoconstriction but may cause respiratory depression and exacerbation of hypoxemia and hypercapnia.
7. If these measures prove ineffective—
   a. Inotropic agents may be required to augment cardiac output, particularly in hypotensive patients.
   b. Insertion of an intra-aortic balloon pump can be very beneficial in patients with acute cardiogenic pulmonary edema, especially when secondary to myocardial ischemia.
8. The patient should be kept on strict bed rest with continuous monitoring of cardiac rhythm, BP, and pulse oximetry.

Q.80. What are the X-ray findings of pulmonary edema?

Ans. The X-ray findings of pulmonary edema are:
- Upper lobe diversion
- Kerley's B line
- Bilateral hilar opacities (Bat's wing appearance)
- Pleural effusion.

Q.81. Define heart failure.

Ans. Heart failure is the clinical syndrome that develops when the heart cannot maintain an adequate cardiac output, or can do so only at the expense of an elevated filling pressure.

Q.82. What are the types of heart failure?

Ans. The types of heart failure:

i. According to onset—

  - Acute heart failure
  - Chronic heart failure
  - Acute on chronic heart failure.
- ii. According to involvement—
  - Left heart failure
  - Right heart failure
  - Biventricular heart failure.
- iii. According to function—
  - Systolic dysfunction
  - Diastolic dysfunction.
- iv. According to cardiac output—
  - High output failure
  - Low output failure.

Q.83. What are the common causes of heart failure?

Ans. The common causes of heart failure are:
- Myocardial infarction
- Myocarditis/cardiomyopathy
- Hypertension
- Aortic stenosis
- Mitral stenosis
- Ventricular septal defect
- Atrial fibrillation.

Q.84. What are the factors that may precipitate or aggravate heart failure?

Ans. The factors are:
- Myocardial ischemia or infarction.
- Intercurrent illness, e.g. infection.
- Arrhythmia, e.g. atrial fibrillation.
- Inappropriate reduction of therapy.
- Administration of a drug with negative inotropic properties (e.g. β-blocker) or fluid-retaining properties (e.g. nonsteroidal anti-inflammatory drugs (NSAIDs) and corticosteroids).
- Pulmonary embolism.
- Conditions associated with increased metabolic demand, e.g. pregnancy, thyrotoxicosis, and anemia.
- IV fluid overload, e.g. postoperative IV infusion.

Q.85. What are the causes of right heart failure?

Ans. The causes of right heart failure are:
- Secondary to left heart failure

- Chronic lung disease (cor pulmonale)
- Multiple pulmonary emboli
- Pulmonary valvular stenosis.

Q.86. What are the clinical signs of right ventricular hypertrophy?

Ans. The clinical signs of right ventricular hypertrophy are epigastric pulsation and left parasternal heave.

Q.87. What is cor pulmonale?

Ans. Right ventricular hypertrophy with or without failure due to pulmonary vascular lung parenchyma or chest wall cause.

Q.88. What are the causes of tender hepatomegaly?

Ans. The causes of tender hepatomegaly are:

- Congestive cardiac failure
- Viral hepatitis
- Liver abscess
- Hepatoma
- Budd-Chiari syndrome.

Q.89. What are the cardinal features (typical signs) of right heart failure?

Ans. The cardinal features of right heart failure are:

- Peripheral pitting edema
- Raised JVP
- Enlarged tender liver.

Q.90. What are the cardinal features of left heart failure?

Ans. The cardinal features of left heart failure are:

- Paroxysmal nocturnal dyspnea
- Orthopnea
- Cold perspiration
- Pulsus alternans
- Gallop rhythm
- Bilateral basal crepitations altered after coughing.

Q.91. What are the complications of heart failure?

Ans. The complications of heart failure are:

- Renal failure
- Hypokalemia
- Hyperkalemia
- Hyponatremia
- Thromboembolism
- Arrhythmias—Atrial and ventricular.

Q.92. How can you treat a case of chronic heart failure?

Ans. i. General measures:
- Education—Explanation of nature of disease, treatment, and self-help strategies.
- Diet—Good general nutrition and weight reduction for the obese. Avoidance of high-salt foods and added salt, especially for patients with severe congestive heart failure.
- Smoking cessation.
- Exercise—Regular moderate aerobic exercise within limits of symptoms.
- Alcohol—Alcohol moderation or elimination of alcohol consumption. Alcohol-induced cardio-myopathy requires abstinence.
- Vaccination—Influenza and pneumococcal vaccination should be considered.

ii. Drug therapy:
- Diuretic therapy—Furosemide and spironolactone, usually in combination.
- Vasodilator therapy—Nitrates reduce preload as venodilators and hydralazine reduce afterload as arterial dilators.
- Angiotensin-converting enzyme (ACE) inhibitor therapy—Lisinopril and ramipril.
- Angiotensin receptor blocker (ARB) therapy—Losartan and valsartan.
- β-adrenoceptor blocker therapy—Bisoprolol and metoprolol.
- Digoxin and amiodarone.

iii. Coronary revascularization.

iv. Heart transplantation.

Q.93. What are the drugs used in heart failure?

Ans.
- Diuretic therapy—Furosemide and spironolactone usually in combination.
- Vasodilator therapy—Nitrates reduce preload and arterial dilators, such as hydralazine, reduce afterload.
- Angiotensin-converting enzyme (ACE) inhibition therapy—Lisinopril and ramipril.
- Angiotensin receptor blocker (ARB) therapy—Losartan and valsartan.
- β-adrenoceptor blocker therapy—Bisoprolol and metoprolol.
- Digoxin and amiodarone.

Q.94. Describe the mechanism of ACE inhibitors in heart failure.

Ans. ACE inhibitor interrupts the vicious circle of neurohumoral activation that is characteristic of moderate and severe heart failure by preventing the conversion of angiotensin I to angiotensin II, thereby preventing salt and water retention, peripheral arterial and venous vasoconstriction, and activation of the sympathetic nervous system.

Q.95. What are the contraindications of ACE inhibitor?

Ans. The contraindications of ACE inhibitor are pregnancy, bilateral renal artery stenosis, and hyperkalemia.

Q.96. What are the contraindications of β-blocker?

Ans. The contraindications of β-blocker are bronchial asthma, COPD, heart block, and peripheral vascular disease.

Q.97. What is the role of digoxin in heart failure?

Ans. There is little role of digoxin in heart failure if the patient is in sinus rhythm but improves heart failure if atrial fibrillation is present.

Q.98. Which drug has survival benefit in heart failure?

Ans. Spironolactone has survival benefit in heart failure.

Q.99. What are the causes of generalized edema?

Ans. The causes of generalized edema are:

- Cardiac failure—Right or combined left and right heart failure.
- Chronic venous insufficiency—Varicose veins,
- Hypoalbuminemia: Nephrotic syndrome, chronic liver disease, and protein-losing enteropathy.
- Drugs:
  - NSAIDs
  - Amlodipine.
- Idiopathic:
  - Women > men.
- Chronic lymphatic obstruction.

Q.100. What are the causes of unilateral leg swelling?

Ans. The causes of unilateral leg swelling are:

- Deep vein thrombosis
- Lymphedema
- Cellulitis
- Calf hematoma
- Rupture of Baker's cyst.

Q.101. What are the causes of nonpitting edema?

Ans. The causes of nonpitting edema are:
- Lymphedema
- Myxedema (hypothyroidism).

Q.102. Define palpitation.

Ans. Palpitation is the subjective awareness of the heartbeat.

Q.103. What are the causes of palpitation?

Ans. The causes of palpitations are:
- Irregular—Atrial fibrillation and ectopics.
- Regular—Paroxysmal—SVT/ VT.
- Sustained—Sinus tachycardia, anemia, anxiety, and valve disease.

Q.104. What is sinus tachycardia?

Ans. Sinus rate more than 100 beats per minute is sinus tachycardia.

Q.105. Tell some common causes of sinus tachycardia?

Ans. Some common causes of sinus tachycardia are:
- Anxiety
- Fever
- Anemia
- Heart failure
- Thyrotoxicosis.

Drugs—e.g. β-agonists (salbutamol).

Q.106. What is sinus bradycardia?

Ans. Sinus rate<60 beats per minute.

Q.107. Tell some common causes of sinus bradycardia?

Ans. Some common causes of sinus bradycardia are:
- MI (especially inferior MI)
- Hypothyroidism
- Obstructive jaundice
- Raised intracranial pressure.

Drugs—e.g. β-blockers, digoxin, and verapamil.

Q.108. What is the most common arrhythmia?

Ans. Atrial fibrillation is the most common arrhythmia.

Q.109. What is the character of pulse in atrial fibrillation?

Ans. Irregularly irregular pulse.

Q.110. What are the causes of irregularly irregular pulse?

Ans. The causes of irregularly irregular pulse are:
- Atrial fibrillation

- Multiple ectopics
- Atrial flutter with variable block.

Q.111. Tell five common causes of atrial fibrillation?

Ans. The five common causes of atrial fibrillation are:
- Chronic rheumatic heart disease, particularly mitral stenosis
- Ischemic heart disease
- Hypertension
- Thyrotoxicosis
- Lone atrial fibrillation.

Q.112. What are the common presentations of atrial fibrillation?

Ans. The common presentations of atrial fibrillation are:
- Palpitation
- Heart failure
- Thromboembolism, e.g. stroke.

Q.113. What are the types of atrial fibrillation?

Ans. i. According to duration—
- Paroxysmal
- Persistent
- Permanent.

ii. According to heart rate—
- Fast atrial fibrillation—Ventricular rate is >100/minute
- Slow atrial fibrillation—Ventricular rate is <100/minute.

Q.114. What will you get by examining this patient with atrial fibrillation?

Ans. We get by examining patients with atrial fibrillation are:
- Irregularly irregular pulse
- Pulsus deficit
- Absence of a-wave in JVP
- Variable intensity of first heart sound.

Q.115. What are the ECG findings in atrial fibrillation?

Ans. The ECG findings are:
- Absence of P-wave
- Presence of fibrillatory f-wave
- R-waves are irregular in space and amplitude.

Q.116. Tell the outline of management of atrial fibrillation?

Ans. The outline of management are:
- Restoration of sinus rhythm (either by drug or DC shock)

- Maintenance of sinus rhythm
- Control of heart rate during atrial fibrillation
- Prevention of thromboembolism (either by warfarin or aspirin)
- Treatment of underlying cause.

Q.117. How can you assess risk of thromboembolism in atrial fibrillation?

Ans. By using the CHADS score:

- Congestive heart failure (1 point)
- Hypertension (1 point)
- Age > 75 (1 point)
- Diabetes mellitus (1 point)
- Stroke or transient ischemic attack (2 points)

Score: 0 = aspirin therapy only, 1= warfarin or aspirin, and ≥ 2 = warfarin.

Q.118. What is the role of digoxin in atrial fibrillation?

Ans. Digoxin controls heart rate but cannot convert atrial fibrillation to sinus rhythm.

Q.119. What is lone atrial fibrillation? How will you manage the patient?

Ans. Atrial fibrillation having no cause and patient have structurally normal heart is known as 'lone atrial fibrillation'.

This patient needs no anticoagulation because of low-risk of thromboembolism. Aspirin may be used.

Q.120. A 25-year-old young woman presents with palpitation for half an hour with no other complaints. On examination pulse is 165/minute regular, no other abnormality. What is your diagnosis?

Ans. The diagnosis is supraventricular tachycardia.

Q.121. How will you treat this patient?

Ans. We treat this patient by:

- Confirmation of diagnosis by ECG
- Reassurance
- Vagotonic maneuver, e.g. carotid sinus massage and Valsalva maneuver
- Sedation by diazepam
- Drugs—IV adenosine, verapamil, and β-blocker
- DC cardioversion if cardiac decompensation.

Q.122. What is the contraindication of IV adenosine?

Ans. Bronchial asthma is the contraindication of IV adenosine.

Q.123. What is syncope?

Ans. Syncope is the transient loss of consciousness due to reduced cerebral perfusion.

Q.124. What are the causes of syncope?

Ans. The causes of syncope are:

i. Cardiac diseases:
   - Arrhythmia
     - Bradyarrhythmia and tachyarrhythmia.
   - Mechanical—
     - Ischemic LV dysfunction
     - Aortic stenosis
     - Hypertrophic obstructive cardiomyopathy.

ii. Inappropriate vasodilatation:
   - Simple faint
   - Malignant vasovagal syndrome
   - Postural hypotension
   - Situational syncope, e.g. cough syncope, and micturation syncope.

iii. Neurogenic syncope:
   - Epilepsy
   - Transient ischemic attack.

iv. Metabolic—Hypoglycemia.

Q.125. What is Stokes-Adams attacks?

Ans. Recurrent syncope due to episodes of ventricular asystole is called Stokes-Adams attacks.

Q.126. What are the causes of Stokes-Adams attacks?

Ans. The causes of Stokes-Adams attacks are:

- Complete heart block
- Mobitz type II second-degree AV block
- Sinoatrial disease.

Q.127. What is Stokes-Adams syndrome?

Ans. Stokes-Adams attacks due to complete heart block.

Q.128. What are the features of complete heart block?

Ans. The features of complete heart block are:

- It may be asymptomatic or recurrent syncope (Stokes-Adams attacks)
- Bradycardia—Slow (25–50/min) and regular large-volume pulse
- Intermittent cannon waves in JVP
- Variable intensity of first heart sound.

Q.129. What are the causes of complete heart block?

Ans. The causes of complete heart block are:

i. Congenital
ii. Acquired
- Idiopathic fibrosis
- MI/ischemia
- Inflammation
- Acute—Aortic root abscess in infective endocarditis
- Chronic—Sarcoidosis and Chagas disease.
- Cardiac surgery
- Drugs—Digoxin and β-blocker.

Q.130. What are the ECG findings of complete heart block?

Ans. The findings are:
- Complete AV dissociation
- Slow ventricular rate (25–50/min)
- PR interval variable but PP interval and RR interval fixed.

Q.131. What is the treatment of chronic complete heart block?

Ans. Permanent pacemaker is the treatment of chronic complete heart block whether symptomatic or asymptomatic.

Q.132. A 75-year-old male gives a history of loss of consciousness yesterday. His wife says he lost consciousness while he was sitting in a chair; he became pale but regained consciousness within few seconds with facial flushing. What is your diagnosis?

Ans. The diagnosis is cardiac syncope.

Q.133. How can you differentiate cardiac syncope from simple faint (vasovagal syncope)?

Ans.

	Cardiac syncope	Neurocardiogenic syncope (vasovagal syncope)
Premonitory symptoms	Often none	Nausea
	Light-headedness Palpitation Chest pain	Light-headedness Sweating
Unconscious period	Extreme 'death-like' pallor	Pallor
Recovery	Rapid recovery (< 1 min) Flushing	Slow Nausea Light-headedness

Q.134. How can you differentiate cardiac syncope from seizures?

Ans.

	Cardiac syncope	Seizures
Premonitory symptoms	Often none	Confusion
	Light-headedness Palpitation	Hyperexcitability Olfactory hallucinations
	Chest pain Breathlessness	'Aura'
Unconscious period	Extreme 'death-like' pallor	Prolonged (> 1 min) unconsciousness Motor seizure activity Tongue-biting Urinary incontinence
Recovery	Rapid recovery (< 1 min) Flushing	Prolonged confusion (> 5 min) Headache Focal neurological signs

Q.135. Define hypertension.

Ans. Persistent rise of blood pressure above the normal is called hypertension.

Or

The level of blood pressure at which the benefits of treatment outweigh its costs and hazards is called hypertension.

Q.136. What are the objectives of the initial evaluation of a patient with high BP readings?

Ans. The objectives are:
- To obtain accurate and representative measurements of BP.
- To identify contributory factors and any underlying cause (secondary hypertension).
- To assess other risk factors and quantify cardiovascular risk.
- To detect any complications (target organ damage) that are already present.
- To identify comorbidity that may influence the choice of antihypertensive therapy.

Q.137. What are the causes of hypertension?

Ans. The causes of hypertension are:

- Essential hypertension > 95%
- Secondary hypertension <5%.

Q.138. What are the secondary causes?

Ans. Secondary causes are:

- Renal disease:
  - Renal vascular disease—Renal artery stenosis
  - Parenchymal renal disease, particularly glomerulonephritis
  - Polycystic kidney disease.
- Endocrine disease:
  - Pheochromocytoma
  - Cushing's syndrome
  - Primary hyperaldosteronism (Conn's syndrome)
  - Acromegaly
  - Primary hypothyroidism
  - Thyrotoxicosis.
- Drugs:
- Oral contraceptives containing estrogens and corticosteroids
- NSAIDs.
- Coarctation of the aorta
- Alcohol
- Obesity
- Pregnancy (pre-eclampsia).

Q.139. What is the most common cause of hypertension?

Ans. The most common cause of hypertension is ideopathic.

Q.140. What is the second common cause of hypertension?

Ans. The second common cause of hypertension are renal diseases.

Q.141. Classify hypertension.

Ans. Classification according to JNC VII.

BP classification	SBP mmHg		DBP mmHg
Normal	<120	and	<80
Prehypertension	120–139	or	80–89
Stage 1 Hypertension	140–159	or	90–99
Stage 2 Hypertension	≥160	or	≥100

Q.142. What are the target organs of hypertension?

Ans. The target organs of hypertension are:
- Central nervous system
- Eyes
- Heart
- Kidneys
- Blood vessels.

Q.143. What are the CNS complications of hypertension?

Ans. The CNS complications of hypertension are:
- Hypertensive encephalopathy
- Transient ischemic attack
- Stroke
- Subarachnoid hemorrhage.

Q.144. What are the eye complications of hypertension?

Ans. 1. Hypertensive retinopathy
   - Grade 1—Arteriolar thickening, tortuosity, and increased reflectiveness (silver wiring).
   - Grade 2—Grade 1 plus constriction of veins at arterial crossings (arteriovenous nipping).
   - Grade 3—Grade 2 plus evidence of retinal ischemia (flame-shaped or blot hemorrhages and 'cotton wool' exudates).
   - Grade 4—Grade 3 plus papilledema.
2. Central retinal vein thrombosis.

Q.145. How can you measure blood pressure?

Ans. Blood pressure is measured in the following ways:
- Use a machine that has been validated, well-maintained, and properly calibrated.
- Measure sitting BP routinely, with additional standing BP in elderly and diabetic patients and those with possible postural hypotension.
- Remove tight clothing from the arm.
- Support the arm at the level of the heart.
- Use a cuff of appropriate size (the bladder must encompass > two-thirds of the arm).
- Lower the pressure slowly (2 mmHg/sec).
- Read the BP to the nearest 2 mmHg.
- Use phase V (disappearance of sounds) to measure diastolic BP.
- Take two measurements at each visit.

Q.146. Outline the treatment strategy of treatment of hypertension.

Ans. 1. General measures—
- Lifestyle modifications to manage hypertension.

2. Antihypertensive drugs.
3. Treatment of underlying cause in secondary hypertension.

Modification	Recommendation
Weight reduction	Maintain normal body weight (body mass index is 18.5–24.9 kg/m^2).
Adopt DASH eating plan 1	Consume a diet rich in fruits, vegetables, and low-fat dairy products with a reduced content of saturated and total fat
Dietary sodium reduction	Reduce dietary sodium intake to no more than 100 mmol per day (2.4 gm sodium or 6 gm sodium chloride)
Physical activity	Engage in regular aerobic physical activity such as brisk walking (at least 30 min per day, most days of the week)
Moderation of alcohol	Limit consumption to no more than consumption 2 drinks per day in most men and to no more than 1 drink per day in women

Q.147. What is DASH?

Ans. DASH means dietary approaches to stop hypertension.

Q.148. Classify antihypertensive drugs.

Ans.
- Thiazides or thiazide-like diuretics
- ACE inhibitors
- Angiotensin II receptor blockers
- Calcium channel blockers
- β-blockers
- Others—α-blocker and centrally acting drugs, e.g. clonidine.

Q.149. What is the goal or target of antihypertensive therapy?

Ans. The goal BP is <140/90 mmHg in otherwise normal individual and

In patients with diabetes or renal disease, the goal BP is <130/80 mmHg.

Q.150. What is the threshold for antihypertensive drugs?

Ans. Threshold for offering drug treatment—
- BP > 160/100 mm Hg
- Isolated systolic hypertension (systolic BP> 160 mmHg)
- BP > 140/90 mmHg and target organ damage or 10 years CVD 20%.

Q.151. What are the strategies of antihypertensive drug combination?

Ans.

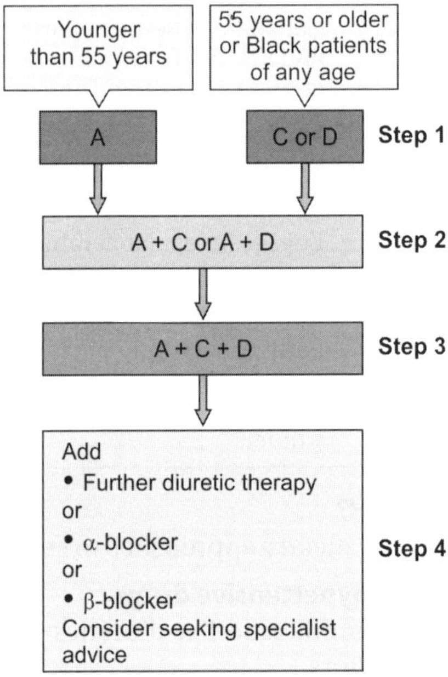

(A = ACE inhibitor (consider angiotensin II receptor antagonist if ACE-intolerant); C = calcium channel blocker; D = thiazide-type diuretic).

Q.152. Which drug will you choose to treat hypertension in pregnancy?

Ans. Calcium channel blocker and methyldopa.

Q.153. What is hypertensive encephalopathy?

Ans. Hypertensive encephalopathy is an acute and transient disturbance of cerebral function due to sudden rise of blood pressure.

Q.154. What are the clinical features of hypertensive encephalopathy?

Ans. The clinical features of hypertensive encephalopathy are:

- Abrupt onset
- Slurring of speech
- Blurring of vision
- Paresthesia
- Papilledema
- Disorientation
- Convulsion
- Coma.

Q.155. What is malignant hypertension?

Ans. Malignant hypertension is a syndrome associated with an abrupt increase of blood pressure in a patient with underlying hypertension or related to the sudden onset of hypertension in a previously normotensive individual. The absolute level of blood pressure is not as important as its rate of rise.

Clinically, the syndrome is recognized by progressive retinopathy (arteriolar spasm, hemorrhages, exudates, and papilledema), deteriorating renal function with proteinuria, microangiopathic hemolytic anemia, and encephalopathy.

Q.156. What are hypertensive emergency and urgency?

Ans. Hypertensive emergency is the situation when BP should be lowered within 1 hour to reduce morbidity or death, e.g. hypertensive encephalopathy, aortic dissection and MI, etc.

Hypertensive urgency is the situation when BP should be lowered within few hours, e.g. asymptomatic severe hypertension.

Q.157. What is gestational hypertension? What is time limit?

Ans. Elevated blood pressure during pregnancy or first 24 hour postpartum in the absence of previous chronic persistent hypertension or proteinuria.

Q.158. Which type of lipid profile should be preferable?

Ans. Fasting lipid profile.

Q.159. What is white coat hypertension? What is advice with white coat hypertension?

Ans. An unrepresentative surge in BP when measured in the clinic, particularly by a doctor has been termed 'white coat' hypertension.

The risk of cardiovascular disease in these patients is less than that in patients with sustained hypertension but greater than that in normotensive subjects. So these patients should be under regular follow-up.

Q.160. A 9-year-old boy came with the history of fever for 10 days and painful swelling of large joints. He gave a history of sore throat 3 weeks back. On precordium auscultation a soft systolic murmur is found. What is your diagnosis?

Ans. Acute rheumatic fever.

Q.161. What is the pathogenesis of rheumatic fever?

Ans. The condition is triggered by an immune-mediated delayed response to infection with specific strains of group A β-hemolytic streptococci due to antigenic molecular mimicry.

Q.162. Which age group is more vulnerable?

Ans. Age 5–15 years.

Q.163. Which pattern of arthritis occurs in rheumatic fever?

Ans. Migratory polyarthritis.

Q.164. How can you diagnose acute rheumatic fever?

Ans. The diagnosis, made using the revised Jones criteria, is based upon two or more major manifestations, or one major and two or more minor manifestations, along with evidence of preceding streptococcal infection.

Q.165. What are the major criteria?

Ans. The major criteria are:

- Carditis
- Polyarthritis
- Chorea
- Erythema marginatum
- Subcutaneous nodules.

Q.166. What are the minor criteria?

Ans. The minor criteria are:

- Fever

- Arthralgia
- Previous rheumatic fever
- Raised ESR or CRP
- Leukocytosis
- First-degree AV block.

Q.167. What are the supporting evidences of preceding streptococcal infection?

Ans. The supporting evidences of preceding streptococcal infection—

- Recent scarlet fever
- Raised antistreptolysin O or other streptococcal antibody titer
- Positive throat culture.

Q.168. How can you treat acute rheumatic fever?

Ans. **Management of the acute attack**

i. Antibiotic therapy: A single dose of benzathine penicillin 1.2 million U IM or oral phenoxymethylpenicillin 250 mg 6-hourly for 10 days to eliminate any residual streptococcal infection.

   If the patient is penicillin-allergic, erythromycin or a cephalosporin.

ii. Bed rest and supportive therapy: Bed rest till temperature, leukocyte count, and ESR become normal.

iii. Aspirin: 60 mg/kg body weight/day, divided into six doses.

   In adults, 100 mg/kg/day may be needed upto the limits of tolerance or a maximum of 8 gm/day.

   Aspirin should be continued until the ESR has fallen and then gradually tailed off.

iv. Corticosteroids—Indicated in cases with carditis or severe arthritis.

   Prednisolone—1.0–2.0 mg/kg/day in divided doses, should be continued until the ESR is normal, then tailed off.

Secondary prevention

Long-term prophylaxis with penicillin should be given as benzathine penicillin 1.2 million U IM monthly or oral phenoxymethylpenicillin 250 mg 12-hourly upto the age of 21 years or 5 years which is longer.

Q.169. Which valve is most commonly affected in rheumatic fever?

Ans. Mitral valve is most commonly affected in rheumatic fever.

Q.170. What is the most common valvular heart disease?

Ans. Mitral stenosis is the most common heart disease.

Q.171. A 35-year-old female presents with right-sided hemiplegia. On examination you found irregularly irregular pulse, right-sided upper motor neuron lesion and mid-diastolic murmur on heart auscultation. What is your diagnosis?

Ans. CVD (right-sided hemiplegia) due to cerebral embolism as a result of atrial fibrillation from mitral stenosis.

Q.172. What is the most common cause of mitral stenosis?

Ans. The most common cause of mitral stenosis is chronic rheumatic heart disease.

Q.173. What will you get by examining precordium of this patient?

Ans. Inspection—Normal.

Palpation—Tapping apex beat, may have diastolic thrill in the apex. Left parasternal heave and palpable P_2 if pulmonary hypertension.

- Auscultation—Loud S_1 localized low-pitched rough rumbling mid-diastolic murmur best heard in left lateral position with bell of the stethoscope breath-holding after expiration.
- Loud P_2 if pulmonary hypertension.

Q.174. What are the causes of MDM?

Ans. The causes of MDM are:

- Mitral stenosis
- Tricuspid stenosis
- Carey Coombs murmur
- Austin Flint murmur
- Left atrial myxoma.

Q.175. How can you treat mitral stenosis?

Ans. i. Medical:

- Lifelong penicillin either oral or IM for secondary rheumatic prophylaxis.
- Antibiotic prophylaxis for infective endocarditis when necessary.
- Diuretic if heart failure.

- Digoxin if atrial fibrillation.
- Aspirin or warfarin if atrial fibrillation.

ii. Surgical:
- CMC or OMC
- PTMC
- Valve replacement.

Q.176. What are the typical signs of AR?

Ans. The typical signs of AR—
- Pulse—High volume collapsing pulse
- BP—High systolic, low diastolic, and wide pulse pressure
- Thursting apex beat
- Early diastolic murmur on auscultation best heard in left parasternal area in sitting position breath-holding after expiration.

Q.177. Define infective endocarditis.

Ans. This is due to microbial infection of a heart valve (native or prosthetic), the lining of a cardiac chamber or blood vessel, or a congenital anomaly (e.g. septal defect).

Q.178. What are the types of infective endocarditis?

Ans. The types of endocarditis are:
- Acute infective endocarditis
- Subacute infective endocarditis
- Postoperative infective endocarditis.

Q.179. What are the common organisms involved in infective endocarditis?

Ans.
1. Streptococcus— Viridens group and enterococci.
2. Staphylococcus—*Staphylococcus aureus* and coagulase negative
3. Gram-negative bacilli—*Haemophilus* anaerobes
4. Others—Rickettsiae and fungi.

Q.180. What are the peripheral stigmata of infective endocarditis?

Ans. The peripheral stigmata of infective endocarditis are:
- Clubbing
- Splinter hemorrhage
- Osler's nodes
- Janeway lesions
- Purpura
- Roth's spots.

Q.181. Tell the emperical therapy of infective endocarditis?

Ans. Acute—Flucloxacillin and gentamicin.

Subacute or indolent—Benzyl penicillin and gentamicin.

In those with penicillin allergy, a prosthetic valve or suspected methicillin-resistant *Staph. aureus* (MRSA) Infection—Triple therapy with vancomycin, gentamicin, and oral rifampicin.

Q.182. Please name some congenital heart diseases.

Ans. Some congenital heart diseases are:

- ASD(atrial septal defect)
- VSD(ventricular septal defect)
- PDA(patent ductus arteriosus)
- TOF(tetralogy of Fallot)
- Pulmonary stenosis
- Coarctation of aorta
- Aortic stenosis
- Complete transposition of great arteries.

Q.183. Which are cyanotic congenital heart diseases?

Ans. Cyanotic congenital heart diseases are:

- TOF (tetralogy of Fallot)
- Complete transposition of great arteries.

Q.184. Which are acyanotic congenital heart diseases?

Ans. The followings are acyanotic congenital heart diseases—

- ASD(atrial septal defect)
- VSD(ventricular septal defect)
- PDA(patent ductus arteriosus)
- Pulmonary stenosis
- Coarctation of aorta
- Aortic stenosis.

Q.185. Which is the most common congenital heart disease?

Ans. Ventricular septal defect is the most common congenital heart disease.

Q.186. What are the components of TOF?

Ans. The components of TOF are:

- VSD
- Overriding of aorta
- Pulmonary stenosis
- Right ventricular hypertrophy.

Q.187. What are the presentations of TOF?

Ans. The presentation of TOF are:

- Cyanotic spells, e.g. cyanosis during crying, running, and feeding.
- Stunted growth.
- Syncope.

Q.188. What are the findings on examination?

Ans. The findings of examinations are:

- Short stature
- Clubbing
- Cyanosis
- An ejection systolic murmur in pulmonary area.

Q.189. What is the chest X-ray findings of Fallot's tetralogy and ASD?

Ans.
- X-ray findings of TOF are boot-shaped heart and oligemic lung field.
- X-ray findings of ASD are cardiomegaly with fullness of pulmonary conus and plethoric lung field.

Q.190. What is oligemic and plethoric lung field?

Ans. Oligemic lung field means reduced pulmonary vascularities; hence it is more translucent than expected. Plethoric lung field means increased pulmonary blood flow.

Q.191. What is the medical management of TOF?

Ans.
i. During cyanotic spell:
   - Patient should be put in squatting position
   - High flow O_2
   - IV morphine
   - IV β-blocker.

ii. Between cyanotic spell:
   - Oral β-blocker.

Q.192. What are the auscultatory findings of ASD and VSD?

Ans.
- ASD—Ejection systolic murmur in pulmonary area
- VSD—Pansystolic murmur in left parasternal area.

Q.193. What are the clinical presentations of VSD?

Ans. Patient may present as—

a. Cardiac failure in infants.

b. As a murmur with only minor hemodynamic disturbance in older children or adults.

c. Rarely as Eisenmenger's syndrome.

Q.194. What are the physical signs and auscultatory findings in VSD?

Ans. Physical signs and auscultatory findings in VSD are:

- Heaving apex beat
- Left parasternal systolic thrill
- Pansystolic murmur in left sternal edge radiating over whole precordium.

Q.195. What are the causes of acute pericarditis?

Ans. The causes of acute pericarditis are:

- Viral (e.g. Coxsackie B but often not identified)
- Acute MI
- Tuberculosis
- Rheumatic fever
- Connective tissue disease (e.g. SLE)
- Uremia
- Malignant disease.

Q.196. What are the clinical features of acute pericarditis?

Ans. The clinical features of acute pericarditis are:

- Retrosternal chest pain—It radiates to the shoulders and neck, and aggravated by deep breathing, movement, a change of position, exercise and swallowing.
- Pericardial rub.

Q.197. What is cardiomyopathy?

Ans. Cardiomyopathy is defined as "a heterogeneous group of diseases of the myocardium associated with mechanical and/or electrical dysfunction that usually (but not invariably) exhibit inappropriate ventricular hypertrophy or dilatation and are due to a variety of causes that frequently are genetic".

Q.198. What are the types of cardiomyopathies?

Ans. The types of cardiomyopathies are:

- Dilated cardiomyopathy
- Hypertrophic cardiomyopathy
- Restrictive cardiomyopathy
- Arrhythmogenic right ventricular cardiomyopathy
- Obliterative cardiomyopathy.

CHAPTER 2

Respiratory System

Q.1. What are the common presentations (symptoms) of respiratory diseases?

Ans. The common presentations of respiratory diseases are:

- Cough
- Sputum
- Wheeze
- Breathlessness
- Chest pain
- Hemoptysis.

Q.2. What are the causes of cough?

Ans. Causes of cough

i. Acute cough (<3 weeks)
   - Viral respiratory tract infection (rhinitis/sinusitis)
   - Bacterial infection (acute bronchitis)
   - Inhaled foreign body
   - Pneumonia
   - Acute extrinsic allergic alveolitis.

ii. Chronic cough (>8 weeks)
   - COPD
   - Asthma
   - Tuberculosis
   - Lung carcinoma
   - Bronchiectasis
   - Interstitial lung disease.
   - GERD
   - Postviral bronchial hyper-reactivity
   - Rhinitis/sinusitis
   - Cigaret smoking
   - Drugs, especially ACE inhibitors.

Q.3. What are the 'Red flag' symptoms associated with cough ?

Ans. The 'Red flag' symptoms are:
- Hemoptysis
- Breathlessness
- Fever
- Chest pain
- Weight loss.

Q.4. What are the causes of cough with normal chest X-ray?

Ans. The causes are:
- GERD
- Asthma
- Postviral bronchial hyper-reactivity
- Rhinitis/sinusitis
- Cigaret smoking
- Drugs, especially ACE inhibitors
- Viral respiratory tract infection
- Bacterial infection (acute bronchitis)
- Inhalation of irritant dusts/fumes.

Q.5. What are the causes of cough with normal chest examination?

Ans. The causes are:
- GERD
- Cough variant asthma
- Postnasal drip (rhinitis/sinusitis)
- ACE inhibitors.

Q.6. What are the causes of productive cough?

Ans. The causes of productive cough are:
- Pneumonia
- Bronchiectasis
- Lung abscess
- Acute pulmonary edema
- Chronic bronchitis/COPD
- Cystic fibrosis
- Alveolar cell cancer.

Q.7. What are the causes of purulent sputum?

Ans. The causes of purulent sputum are:
- Pneumonia
- Bronchiectasis

- Lung abscess
- COPD (infective exacerbation)
- Cystic fibrosis.

Q.8. What are the causes of copious amount of sputum?

Ans. The causes of copious amount of sputum are:
- Bronchiectasis
- Rupture of a lung abscess or empyema into the bronchial tree
- Pulmonary edema
- Alveolar cell cancer.

Q.9. What is the cause of rusty sputum?

Ans. Pneumococcal pneumonia is the cause of rusty sputum.

Q.10. What are the causes of frothy sputum?

Ans. The causes of forthy sputum are:
- Pulmonary edema
- Alveolar cell carcinoma.

Q.11. What are the causes of wheeze?

Ans. The causes of wheeze are:
- Asthma
- COPD.

Q.12. What is wheeze?

Ans. Musical sound produced by obstruction of small bronchus and bronchioles.

Q.13. What is stridor?

Ans. Sound produced by obstruction of large bronchus whether intrathoracic or extrathoracic.

Q.14. What are the causes of breathlessness according to time frame?

Ans. i. Minutes
- Pulmonary thromboembolism
- Pneumothorax
- Acute left ventricular failure
- Asthma
- Inhaled foreign body.

ii. Hours to days
- Pneumonia
- Asthma
- Exacerbation of COPD.

iii. Weeks to months
  - Anemia
  - Pleural effusion
  - Respiratory neuromuscular disorders.

iv. Months to years
  - COPD
  - Pulmonary fibrosis
  - Pulmonary tuberculosis.

Q.15. What are the causes of chronic breathlessness, according to lung and heart cause?

Ans. **Lung causes are**:
- Chronic obstructive pulmonary disease
- Chronic asthma
- Chronic pulmonary thromboembolism
- Bronchial carcinoma
- Interstitial lung diseases: Sarcoidosis, fibrosing alveolitis, and extrinsic allergic alveolitis.
- Lymphatic carcinomatosis
- Large pleural effusion(s).

Heart causes are:
- Chronic congestive cardiac failure
- Myocardial ischemia.

Q.16. Tell the MRC grading of dyspnea.

Ans. Grade 1—Breathless when hurrying on the level or walking up a slight hill.

Grade 2—Breathless when walking with people of own age or on level ground.

Grade 3—Has to stop because of breathlessness when walking on level ground at own pace.

Q.17. What is hemoptysis?

Ans. Hemoptysis means coughing up blood.

Q.18. What is massive hemoptysis?

Ans. Coughing out 200ml of blood in 24 hours.

Q.19. Tell six common causes of hemoptysis.

Ans. The six common causes of hemoptysis are:
- Tuberculosis
- Bronchial carcinoma
- Bronchiectasis
- Pneumonia
- Mitral stenosis
- Pulmonary infarction.

Q.20. What is pleural effusion?

Ans. The accumulation of serous fluid within the pleural space is termed pleural effusion.

Q.21. Tell the common causes of pleural effusion.

Ans. The common causes of pleural effusion are:

- Pneumonia (parapneumonic effusion)
- Tuberculosis
- Pulmonary infarction
- Malignant disease
- Cardiac failure
- Subdiaphragmatic disorders (subphrenic abscess, pancreatitis, etc).

Q.22. How can you differentiate exudative pleural effusion from transudative pleural effusion?

Ans.

Exudative	Transudative
Protein content > 3 gm/dL	Protein content < 3 gm/dL
Pleural fluid LDH >200 UL/L	Pleural fluid LDH <200 UL/L

Q.23. What is the Light's criteria?

Ans. Light's criteria for distinguishing pleural transudate from exudate

- Pleural fluid is an exudate if one or more of the following criteria are met:
  - Pleural fluid protein: Serum protein ratio > 0.5
  - Pleural fluid LDH: Serum LDH ratio > 0.6
  - Pleural fluid LDH > two-thirds of the upper limit of normal serum LDH.

Q.24. When is Light's criteria applicable?

Ans. When pleural fluid protein is between 2.5 and 3.5 gm/dL.

Q.25. Tell five common causes of exudative pleural effusion.

Ans. The five common causes of exudative pleural effusion are:

- Pneumonia (para-pneumonic effusion)
- Tuberculosis
- Pulmonary infarction
- Malignant disease, e.g. carcinoma of bronchus and lymphoma
- Connective tissue diseases (SLE).

Q.26. Tell five common causes of transudative pleural effusion.

Ans. The five common causes of transudative pleural effusion are:
- Cardiac failure
- Nephrotic syndrome
- Chronic liver disease
- Malnutrition
- Hypothyroidism.

Q.27. What findings will you get by examining the patient with right-sided pleural effusion?

Ans.
- Inspection
  - Movement diminished on right side
- Palpation
  - Trachea and apex beat deviated to left
  - Expansibility reduced on right side
  - Vocal fremitus diminished on right side
- Percussion
  - Stony dull on right side
- Auscultation
  - Breath sound diminished or absent on right side
  - Vocal resonance diminished or absent on right side.

Q.28. How much fluid is to be present to detect clinically and radiologically?

Ans. At least 500 mL clinically and 300 mL radiologically in PA film.

Q.29. What are the purposes of aspiration?

Ans.
- Diagnostic
  - To detect the cause.
- Therapeutic purposes
  - To reduce breathlessness.

Q.30. How much fluid should be drawn in case of diagnosis and therapeutic purposes?

Ans. At least 50 mL for diagnostic purpose and not more than 1.5 L on first occasion.

Q.31. How much fluid will you aspirate on first occasion?

Ans. Not more than 1.5 L.

Q.32. What will happen if you aspirate more than 1.5 L or rapidly?

Ans. Re-expansion pulmonary edema.

Q.33. What are the obstructive pulmonary diseases?

Ans. The obstructive pulmonary diseases are:
- COPD
- Bronchial asthma.

Q.34. What are the restrictive pulmonary diseases?

Ans. The restrictive pulmonary diseases are:
- Interstitial lung disease
- Pulmonary fibrosis.

Q.35. How can you differentiate obstructive from restrictive lung diseases?

Ans.

Test	Obstructive	Restrictive
FEV1	↓↓	↓
VC	↓ or Normal	↓↓
FEV1/VC	↓	Normal or ↑

Q.36. Define COPD.

Ans. COPD is defined as a preventable and treatable lung disease with some significant extrapulmonary effects that may contribute to the severity in individual patients. The pulmonary component is characterized by airflow limitation that is not fully reversible. The airflow limitation is usually progressive and associated with an abnormal inflammatory response of the lung to noxious particles or gases.

Q.37. What are the components of COPD?

Ans. The components of COPD are:
- Chronic bronchitis
- Emphysema.

Q.38. Define chronic bronchitis.

Ans. Chronic bronchitis is defined as cough and sputum on most days for at least 3 consecutive months for at least 2 successive years.

Q.39. Define emphysema.

Ans. Emphysema is defined as abnormal permanent enlargement of the airspaces distal to the terminal bronchioles, accompanied by destruction of their walls and without obvious fibrosis.

Q.40. Define airflow obstruction.

Ans. FEV1< 80% predicted and FEV1: FVC<70%.

Q.41. What are the extrapulmonary manifestations (systemic features) of COPD?

Ans. Extrapulmonary manifestations include impaired nutrition, weight loss and skeletal muscle dysfunction and increased prevalence of osteoporosis.

Q.42. What are the causes of COPD?

Ans. The causes of COPD are:
- Smoking accounts for more than 95% of cases
- Occupational dust and chemicals
- Indoor and outdoor air pollution
- Alpha 1 antitrypsin deficiency.

Q.43. How much smoking accounts for COPD?

Ans. At least 10 pack years (1 pack year = 20 cigarets/day/year).

Q.44. How many smokers are susceptible to develop COPD?

Ans. 15% of smokers are susceptible to develop COPD.

Q.45. What are the common presentations of COPD?

Ans. The common presentations of COPD are:
- Cough with sputum production (smoker's cough)
- Breathlessness.

Q.46. Tell the MRC grading of dyspnea.

Ans.

Grade	Degree of breathlessness related to activities
0	No breathlessness except with strenuous exercise
1	Breathlessness when hurrying on the level or walking up a slight hill
2	Walks slower than contemporaries on level ground because of breathlessness or has to stop for breath when walking at own pace
3	Stops for breath after walking about 100 m or after a few minutes on level ground
4	Too breathless to leave the house, or breathless when dressing or undressing.

Q.47. Is airflow obstruction reversible in COPD?

Ans. Airflow obstruction in emphysema is irreversible but in chronic bronchitis there is some degree of reversibility of airflow obstruction due to presence of inflammation.

Q.48. What are the differences between emphysema and chronic bronchitis?

Ans.

Feature	Chronic bronchitis	Emphysema
Diagnosis	Clinical	Pathological
Appearance	Blue bloater	Pink puffer
Cyanosis	Prominent	Absent
Hyperinflation	+	++
Dyspnea	+	++
Cough	++	+
Cor pulmonale	++	+

A combination of emphysema and bronchitis are found in most patients with COPD.

Q.49. What are the patterns of emphysema?

Ans. Centriacinar, panacinar, and periacinar.

Q.50. What findings can you get by examining this patient?

Ans.
- Patient is dyspneic.
- Pursed-lip breathing.
- Cyanosis.
- Excavation of supraclavicular and suprasternal fossae, indrawing of costal margins, and intercostals spaces.
- Contraction of sternomastoid and scalene muscles on inspiration.
- Tracheal tug.
- Reduced cricosternal distance.
- Barrel chest.
- Loss of cardiac dullness, and lowered down liver dullness.
- Vesicular breath sound with prolonged expiration.
- Low or medium-pitched rhonchi.

Q.51. How can you predict acute infective exacerbation?

Ans. We can predict acute infective exacerbation by—
- Increased breathless and cough
- Increased sputum volume and purulence
- Fever.

Q.52. What are the most common pathogens in acute infective exacerbations?

Ans. *Streptococcus pneumoniae*
Haemophilus influenzae
Moraxella catarrhalis.

Q.53. How would you investigate this patient?

Ans. Investigate by—
- Blood—CBC, ESR
- X-ray chest PA view
- ECG
- ABG
- Sputum—Microscopy and C/S
- Lung function test
- HRCT.

Q.54. Tell the radiological findings in COPD.

Ans. The radiological findings in COPD are:
- Hyperinflated lung field
- Low flat diaphragm
- Long tubular heart shadow
- Hyperlucent lung fields
- Horizontal ribs
- Widened intercostal spaces
- Roomy apex
- Bullae.

Q.55. What may be the ECG findings in COPD?

Ans. The ECG findings in COPD are:
- Right ventricular hypertrophy +/– strain
- Right atrial hypertrophy (P pulmonale)
- Multifocal atrial tachycardia.

Q.56. What may be the ABG abnormalities in COPD?

Ans.
- Type II respiratory failure ($PaO_2<8$ and $PaCO_2>6.6$) in chronic bronchitis.
- Type I respiratory failure ($PaO_2<8$ and $PaCO_2<6.6$) in emphysema.

Q.57. Define respiratory failure.

Ans. When pulmonary gas exchange fails to maintain normal arterial oxygen and carbon dioxide levels is termed respiratory failure.

Q.58. What are the types of respiratory failure?

Ans. • Type I and II relates to the absence or presence of hypercapnia (raised $PaCO_2$)
- Type I respiratory failure (PaO_2<8 and $PaCO_2$<6.6)
- Type II respiratory failure (PaO_2<8 and $PaCO_2$>6.6).

Q.59. What are the causes of type I respiratory failure?

Ans. The causes of type I respiratory failure are:
- Acute asthma
- Emphysema
- Pulmonary edema
- Pneumonia
- Lung fibrosis.

Q.60. What are the causes of type II respiratory failure?

Ans. The causes of type II respiratory failure are:
- Acute severe asthma
- COPD
- Ankylosing spondylitis
- Kyphoscoliosis.

Q.61. What are the principles of O_2 therapy in respiratory failure?

Ans. The principles are:
- In type I, high concentration (i.e.>35%, usually 60%)/ high flow (6–8 L/min)
- In type II, low concentration (24%–28%)/low flow(1–2L/min).

Q.62. Why low conc. O_2 is given in COPD with type II respiratory failure?

Ans. A small percentage of patients with severe chronic COPD and type II respiratory failure develop abnormal tolerance to raised $PaCO_2$ and may become dependent on hypoxic drive to breathe. In these patients, lower concentrations of oxygen 24%–28% by Venturi mask should be used to avoid precipitating worsening respiratory depression.

Q.63. Which findings would you expect in lung function tests in COPD?

Ans. FEV1<80% predicted and FEV1: FVC<70% (airflow obstruction)

↑ TLC, FRC and RV

↓ Vital capacity(VC)

↓ TLCO(carbon monoxide transfer factor).

Q.64. Tell me the spirometric staging of COPD.

Ans. Spirometric classification of COPD severity based on postbronchodilator FEV1

Stage	Severity	FEV1
I	Mild	FEV1/FVC < 0.70 FEV1≥80% predicted
II	Moderate	FEV1/FVC < 0.70 50% ≤ FEV1 < 80% predicted
III	Severe	FEV1/FVC < 0.70 30% ≤ FEV1 < 50% predicted
IV	Very severe	FEV1/FVC < 0.70 FEV1 < 30% predicted or FEV1 < 50% predicted plus chronic respiratory failure

Q.65. How can you manage a patient with stable COPD?

Ans. i. General measures—Stop smoking completely and permanently.
- Vaccination for influenza and pneumococcal pneumonia.

ii. Drug therapy—
- **MildCOPD**—Short-acting bronchodilators, such as the β_2-agonists salbutamol or the anticholinergic, ipratropium bromide, as needed.
- **Moderate COPD**—Regular short-acting bronchodilators (alone/combination)

  +

  Longer-acting bronchodilators, such as the β_2-agonists salmeterol and formoterol, or the anticholinergic tiotropium bromide (alone/combination)
- **Severe COPD**—Short-acting bronchodilators (alone/combination)

  +

  Longer-acting bronchodilators, such as the β_2-agonists salmeterol and formoterol, or the anticholinergic tiotropium bromide(alone/combination)

  +

  Inhaled corticosteroids (ICS) if two or more exacerbations requiring antibiotics or oral steroids per year.

  +/–

  Oral theophylline.

Q.66. What are the indications of steroid in COPD?

Ans. Indications of steroid in COPD are:

- Severe disease (FEV1 < 50%) with two or more exacerbations requiring antibiotics or oral steroids per year—ICS.
- Acute exacerbations of COPD—Oral prednisolone, doses of 30 mg/day for 10 days are recommended.

Q.67. What are the surgical treatments for COPD?

Ans. Bullectomy, lung volume reduction surgery (LVRS), and lung transplantation.

Q.68. How would you manage acute exacerbations of COPD?

Ans. i. Home management—Mild to moderate exacerbation by the use of—

- Increased bronchodilator therapy
- A short course of oral corticosteroids
- Antibiotics if appropriate.

ii. Hospitalization—Oxygen 24% or 28%

- Bronchodilators—Nebulized short-acting β_2-agonists combined with an anticholinergic agent (e.g. salbutamol with ipratropium).
- Corticosteroids—Oral prednisolone—30 mg daily for 10 days.
- Antibiotics—Amoxicillin or macrolide.
- Noninvasive ventilation for severe hypercapneic respiratory failure (pH<7.35)
- Respiratory stimulant, i.e. doxapram if noninvasive ventilation is not available.

Q.69. What are the indications for hospitalization?

Ans. The indications for hospitalization are:

- Cyanosis
- Peripheral edema
- An alteration in consciousness
- Comorbidity
- Social isolation.

Q.70. What are the complications of COPD?

Ans. The complications of COPD are:

- Pulmonary hypertension
- Cor pulmonale
- Respiratory failure

- Polycythemia
- Pneumothorax
- Secondary infection.

Q.71. What are the criteria for discharge of COPD patient?

Ans. When the patient is clinically stable on his or her maintenance medication.

Q.72. What is the new method used to assess prognosis of COPD patient?

Ans. BODE index.

Q.73. What is BODE index?

Ans. BODE index is a composite score comprising the body mass index (B), the degree of airflow obstruction (O), a measurement of dyspnea (D) and exercise capacity (E—Distance walked in 6 min (m)).

Q.74. Define cor pulmonale

Ans. Right ventricular hypertrophy with or without failure due to lung parenchyma, vasculature, and chest wall cause.

Q.75. Tell some common causes of cor pulmonale.

Ans. The common causes of cor pulmonale are:

- COPD
- ILD
- Bronchiectasis
- Severe kyphoscoliosis
- Ankylosing spondylitis.

Q.76. Define bronchial asthma.

Ans. Asthma is defined as a chronic inflammatory disorder of the airways, characterized by reversible airflow obstruction causing cough, wheeze, chest tightness, and shortness of breath.

Q.77. How to make diagnosis of asthma?

Ans. Compatible clinical history plus either/or:

FEV1 $\geq$ 15% (and 200 mL) increase following administration of a bronchodilator/trial of corticosteroids > 20% diurnal variation on $\geq$ 3 days in a week for 2 weeks on PEF diary.

FEV1 $\geq$ 15% decrease after 6 mins of exercise.

Q.78. What is the bedside test of asthma?

Ans. Peak expiratory flow rate is the bedside test of asthama.

Q.79. What is reversibility test?

Ans. Reversibility test is to see the reversibility of airflow obstruction in obstructive lung diseases.

Q.80. How is reversibility test done?

Ans. Reversibility test is done by measuring forced expiratory volume in 1 second before and 20 minutes after administration of 200–400 µg of inhaled salbutamol or after 2 weeks of a trial of corticosteroids (e.g. 30 mg prednisolon daily for 2 weeks).

Q.81. When reversibility test is called positive?

Ans. When FEV1 ≥ 15% (or 200 mL) increase following administration of a bronchodilator / trial of corticosteroids.

Q.82. What are the clinical features?

Ans. Typical symptoms include recurrent episodes of wheeze, chest tightness, breathlessness and cough which display a diurnal pattern, with symptoms and lung function being worse in the early morning.

Q.83. How is chronic asthma managed?

Ans. Management of chronic asthma is stepwise to achieve optimum control.

i. **General measures**—
- Patient education about disease process, compliance, inhaler technique, peak flow monitoring, and self-management.
- Avoidance of known precipitants.
- Smoking cessation.
- Immunizations against influenza and pneumococcus.

ii. **Drug therapy**—

Step 1—Occasional use of inhaled short-acting β_2-adrenoreceptor agonist bronchodilators: salbutamol or terbutaline.

Step 2—Inhaled β_2-agonists as required +
- Low dose inhaled corticosteroids (ICS) such as beclomethasone (200–800 µgm/day), budesonide or leukotriene modifier.

Step 3—Inhaled β_2-agonists as required +
- Low dose ICS + long-acting β_2-agonists

Or
- Medium or high dose ICS
  Or
- Low dose inhaled corticosteroids (ICS) + leukotriene modifier.
  Or
- Low dose ICS + sustained release theophylline.

Step 4—Inhaled β_2-agonists as required +
- Medium or high dose ICS + long-acting β_2-agonists
  +/−
- Leukotriene modifier
  +/−
- Sustained release theophylline

Step 5—Step 4 + oral steroid +/− anti-IgE treatment.

Q.84. What is 'rescue' therapy?

Ans. Short courses of oral corticosteroids (prednisolone 30–60 mg daily) are used to regain control of symptoms in mild to moderate exacerbations of bronchial asthma; this is called 'rescue' therapy.

Q.85. What are the indications for 'rescue' courses?

Ans. Indications for 'rescue' courses are:
- Symptoms and PEF progressively worsening day by day
- Fall of PEF below 60% of the patient's personal best recording
- Onset or worsening of sleep disturbance by asthma
- Persistence of morning symptoms until midday
- Progressively diminishing response to an inhaled bronchodilator
- Symptoms severe enough to require treatment with nebulized or injected bronchodilators.

Q.86. When is tapering of the dose of oral steroid necessary to withdraw treatment?

Ans. When it is given for more than 3 weeks.

Q.87. Can you show me how to use inhaler?

Ans. Remove the cap and shake the inhaler. Breathe out gently and place the mouthpiece into the mouth. Incline the head backward to minimize oropharyngeal deposition.

Simultaneously, begin a slow deep inspiration, depress the canister and continue to inhale. Hold the breath for 10 seconds.

Q.88. What are the features of acute severe asthma?

Ans. The features of acute severe asthma are:

- Respiratory rate is ≥ 25/min
- Heart rate is ≥ 110/min
- Inability to complete sentences in 1 breath
- PEF 33%–50% predicted (< 200 L/min).

Q.89. What are the features of life-threatening asthma?

Ans. The features of life-threatening asthma are:

- Cyanosis
- Feeble respiratory effort
- Silent chest
- Bradycardia or arrhythmias
- Hypotension
- Exhaustion
- Confusion
- Coma
- PEF < 33% predicted (< 100 L/min).

Q.90. What is silent chest?

Ans. There is no breath sound heard on auscultation. This is a sign of life-threatening asthma.

Q.91. What are the causes of sudden severe dyspnea?

Ans. The causes of sudden severe dyspnea are:

- Pneumothorax
- Massive pulmonary embolism
- Acute left ventricular failure
- Acute severe asthma
- Inhaled foreign body.

Q.92. How would you manage acute severe asthma?

Ans. We can manage acute severe asthma by the followings—

- Urgent hospitalization and send blood for ABG.
- Nebulized salbutamol 5 mg 2–4 hourly.
- Oxygen — High-flow/60%.
- Prednisolone 40 mg orally (or hydrocortisone 200 mg IV if patient cannot swallow or vomit).
- IV access, chest X-ray, send blood for urea and electrolytes, theophylline level.

- Administer repeat salbutamol 5mg + ipratropium bromide 0.5 mg nebulizer.
- If failure to respond, continuous salbutamol nebulizer 5–10 mg/hr.
- If not respond, consider IV magnesium sulfate 1.2–2 gm over 20 mins, or aminophylline 5 mg/kg loading dose over 20 mins followed by a continuous infusion at 1 mg/kg/hr.
- Correct fluid and electrolytes (esp. K^+)
- Mechanical ventilation if necessary.

Q.93. Which form of salbutamol should be given in acute severe bronchial asthma?

Ans. Nebulized salbutamol.

Q.94. What are the common causes of occupational asthma?

Ans. The common causes of occupational asthma are:
- Isocyanates
- Flour and grain dust
- Colophony and fluxes
- Latex
- Animals
- Aldehydes
- Wood dust.

Q.95. A 45-year-old male presents with cough with profuse amount of sputum for 3 months. What are the possibilities?

Ans. The posibilities are:
- Bronchiectasis, lung abscess, and alveolar cell cancer.

Q.96. What are the causes of foul smelling sputum?

Ans. Bronchiectasis and lung abscess.

Q.97. What is the cause of the fetid sputum?

Ans. Anaerobic infection is the cause of fetid sputum.

Q.98. If anaerobic organism infection, how will you treat the case?

Ans. Treat the case by using metronidazole.

Q.99. Define bronchiectasis.

Ans. Bronchiectasis is the abnormal permanent dilatation of bronchi with destruction of their walls proximal to the terminal bronchioles.

Q.100. What are the common causes of bronchiectasis?

Ans. The common causes of bronchiectasis are:

- Pulmonary tuberculosis
- Pneumonia complicating measles and whooping cough
- Suppurative pneumonia
- Inhaled foreign body
- Congenital—Kartagener's syndrome, cystic fibrosis, and primary hypogammaglobulinemia.

Q.101. What are the components of Kartagener's syndrome?

Ans. Dextrocardia, bronchiectasis, and sinusitis or frontal sinus agenesis.

Q.102. How will you clinically diagnose a case of bronchiectasis?

Ans. Patient presenting with cough with profuse purulent sputum for long time. On examination clubbing and coarse crepitations which alter after coughing.

Q.103. What are the respiratory causes of clubbing?

Ans. The respiratory causes of clubbing are:

- Suppurative lung diseases (lung abscess, bronchiectasis, and empyema thoracis)
- Bronchial carcinoma
- Interstitial lung diseases.

Q.104. What are the cardinal findings on examination in bronchiectasis?

Ans. Clubbing and coarse crepitations which alter after coughing.

Q.105. What will be the color of sputum of pseudomonas infection?

Ans. Greenish sputum.

Q.106. What is the definitive investigation for bronchiectasis?

Ans. High resolution CT scan is the definitive investigation for bronchiectasis.

Q.107. What investigations will you do?

Ans. The investigations are:

- Sputum for bacteriological and mycological examination
- X-ray chest PA view
- HRCT.

Q.108. What are the radiological findings?

Ans. The radiological findings are:
- Linear shadow (tramline)
- Ring shadow
- Multiple small cavities with or without fluid level.

Q.109. How will you treat bronchiectasis?

Ans. Treatments of brochiectasis are:
- Postural drainage— Keeping the affected side up and percuss over the affected part with cupped hand.
- Antibiotic if infection— Amoxicillin commonly used
- Chest physiotherapy.
- Inhaled bronchodilators and corticosteroids if airflow obstruction.
- Surgical treatment— Mobectomy, heart lung transplantation.

Q.110. What is postural drainage?

Ans. Coughing maintaining position of the body to keep affected part of lung up and clab with cupped hand.

Q.111. What is lung abscess?

Ans. Lung abscess is a large localized collection of pus, or a cavity lined by chronic inflammatory tissue, from which pus has escaped by rupture into a bronchus.

Q.112. What is the radiological finding?

Ans. The radiological finding is:
- Cavitary lesion with air-fluid level.

Q.113. How will you treat a lung abscess?

Ans. Treatments of lung abscess are:

i. Postural drainage.
ii. Antibiotic—Amoxicillin plus metronidazole as empirical therapy and change after culture sensitivity result.
iii. Surgical treatment.

Q.114. How long will you give antibiotic?

Ans. 4–6 weeks.

Q.115. A 20-year-old lady presented with fever, right-sided pleuritic chest pain and cough. What is your diagnosis?

Ans. Pneumonia is the diagnosis.

Q.116. Define pneumonia.

Ans. Pneumonia is defined as an acute respiratory illness associated with recently developed radiological pulmonary shadowing which may be segmental, lobar or multilobar.

Pneumonia means inflammation of lung parenchyma.

Q.117. Tell me the clinical classifications of pneumonia.

Ans. Clinical classifications of pneumonia are:
- Community-acquired pneumonia
- Hospital-acquired pneumonia
- Suppurative pneumonia, and aspiration pneumonia
- Pneumonia in immunocompromised hosts.

Q.118. What are the common organisms causing community-acquired pneumonia (CAP)?

Ans. The common organisms are:
- *Streptococcus pneumoniae*
- *Mycoplasma pneumoniae*
- *Legionella pneumophila*
- *Chlamydia pneumoniae*
- *Haemophilus influenzae*
- *Staphylococcus aureus.*

Q.119. What finding will you get on examining the chest?

Ans. **Inspection**—Movement is diminished on affected side.

Palpation—Expansibility reduced on affected side, trachea and apex beat in normal position, vocal fremitus increased on affected side.

Percussion—Woody dull.

Auscultation—Bronchial breath sound and increased vocal resonance.

Q.120. What are the causes of bronchial breath sound?

Ans. The causes of bronchial breath sound are:
- 3Cs
  - Consolidation
  - Cavitation
  - Collapse with patent bronchus
  - Fibrosis.

Q.121. What are the types of breath sound?

Ans. The types of breath sound are:
- Vesicular
- Vesicular with prolonged expiration
- Bronchial.

Q.122. What does 'rusty sputum' indicate?

Ans. It indicates pneumonia due to *Streptococcus pneumoniae.*

Q.123. What investigations will you do?

Ans. Investigations are:

- Blood for TC, DC, ESR and Hb%—Neutrophilic leukocytosis.
- X-ray chest PA view
- Sputum for Gram stain and C/S
- Blood culture
- Pneumococcal antigen detection in serum or urine.

Q.124. When CXR findings will appear in case of pneumonia?

Ans. After 12–18 hours of onset of symptoms.

Q.125. What is the radiological finding in consolidation?

Ans. Homogenous opacity with air bronchogram.

Q.126. When signs of consolidation will appear in pneumonia?

Ans. Usually after 2 days of onset of symptoms.

Q.127. How can you assess severity of pneumonia?

Ans. We can assess severity of pneumonia by using CURB-65 score.

Q.128. What is CURB-65?

Ans. CURB–65 is:

- Confusion
- Urea >7 mmol/L
- Respiratory rate>30/min
- Blood pressure (systolic < 90 mm Hg or diastolic < 60 mmHg)
- Age>65 years (Score 1 point for each feature).

Q.129. What is severe pneumonia?

Ans. Score 3 or more indicates severe pneumonia.

Q.130. How can you treat CAP?

Ans.

i. Oxygen—Maintaining the $PaO_2 \geq 8$ kPa (60 mmHg) or $SaO_2 \geq 92\%$.

ii. Maintain fluid balance.

iii. Antibiotic treatment—Prompt administration of antibiotics improves outcome.

Antibiotic treatment for CAP—

Uncomplicated CAP

- Amoxicillin 500 mg 8-hourly orally or

If patient is allergic to penicillin

- Clarithromycin 500 mg 12-hourly orally or

- Erythromycin 500 mg 6-hourly orally.

If staphylococcus is cultured or suspected

- Flucloxacillin 1–2 gm 6-hourly IV plus
- Clarithromycin 500 mg 12-hourly IV .

Severe CAP

- Clarithromycin 500 mg 12-hourly IV or
- Erythromycin 500 mg 6-hourly IV plus
- Co-amoxiclav 1.2 gm 8-hourly IV or
- Ceftriaxone 1–2 gm daily IV or
- Cefuroxime 1.5 gm 8-hourly IV or
- Amoxicillin 1 gm 6-hourly IV plus flucloxacillin 2 gm 6-hourly IV.

Q.131. What are the complications of pneumonia?

Ans. The complications of pneumonia are:

- Pleural effusion
- Empyema
- Lung abscess
- Hemoptysis
- Pneumothorax
- Distant abscess, e.g. brain abscess
- Septicemia.

Q.132. Define hospital-acquired pneumonia(HAP).

Ans. Hospital-acquired or nosocomial pneumonia refers to a new episode of pneumonia occurring at least 2 days after admission to hospital.

Q.133. What are the organisms involved in hospital-acquired pneumonia(HAP)?

Ans. **In early-onset HAP**—(within 4–5 days of admission), the organisms as CAP

In late-onset HAP—Gram-negative bacteria (e.g. *Escherichia, Pseudomonas* and *Klebsiella* species), *Staphylococcus aureus* (including methicillin-resistant *Staphylococcus aureus* (MRSA)) and anaerobes.

Q.134. How can you treat HAP?

Ans. i. A third-generation cephalosporin (e.g. cefotaxime) with an aminoglycoside (e.g. gentamicin) or meropenem or a monocyclic β-lactam (e.g. aztreonam) and flucloxacillin.

- These antibiotics are all given intravenously, at least initially.

ii. Physiotherapy is important in those who are immobile or old.
iii. Adequate oxygen therapy, fluid support and monitoring are essential.

Q.135. What is aspiration pneumonia?

Ans. Aspiration pneumonia is characterized by destruction of the lung parenchyma by the inflammatory process after the inhalation of septic material during operations on the nose, mouth or throat, under general anesthesia, or of vomitus during anesthesia or coma.

Q.136. What is tuberculosis?

Ans. It is a chronic specific systemic infectious disease caused by *Mycobacterium tuberculosis* complex.

Q.137. What are the organisms causing tuberculosis?

Ans. The organisms are:
- *Mycobacterium tuberculosis*
- *Mycobacterium bovis*
- Atypical mycobacteria, e.g. *M. kansasii, M. marinum,* and *M. avium intracellulare complex.*

Q.138. Tell another mycobacterium other than tuberculosis.

Ans. *Mycobacterium leprae* causing leprosy.

Q.139. Why is mycobacterium called acid or alcohol fast?

Ans. Mycobacterium is called acidor alcohol fast because it resists decolorization with acid and alkali.

Q.140. What are the types of tuberculosis?

Ans. **a. According to site**

i. Pulmonary tuberculosis
- Primary
- Postprimary— Reactivation
  — Reinfection

ii. Extrapulmonary tuberculosis
- Outside the lung parenchyma (according to USA)
- Outside the lung and pleura (according to UK).

b. According to bacteriological specimen

- Smear positive
  - 2 sputum positive for AFB
  - 1 sputum positive with chest X-ray abnormality
  - 1 sputum positive with one culture positive.

- Smear negative
  - Symptoms suggestive of tuberculosis with 3 negative sputum specimens
  - Persisting symptoms after a course of antibiotics
  - 3 negative sputum specimen or repeated X-ray negative.

c. **According to treatment category**
  - Category 1
  - Category 2.

Q.141. What are the sources of infection?

Ans. The sources of infection are:
- Human source
- Bovine source.

Q.142. What are the routes of entry?

Ans. Routes of entry are:
- Nasal (most common)—droplet infection
- Oral
- Percutaneous
- Direct inoculation
- Transplacental.

Q.143. What are the sites of primary tuberculosis?

Ans. The sites of primary tuberculosis are:
- Lungs
- Intestine
- Tonsil.

Q.144. What are the common sites of pulmonary TB?

Ans. The sites of pulmonary TB are:
- Primary pulmonary TB
  - Subpleural lesion.
- Postprimary TB
  - Apical lesion.

Q.145. What are the histological findings in tubercular lesions?

Ans. The histological findings are:
- Caseating granuloma
- Epithelioid cell
- Multinucleated giant cell.

Q.146. What is Ghon's complex?

Ans. A combination of Ghon's focus, hilar lymphadenopathy plus lymphangitis.

Q.147. What is Ghon's focus?

Ans. The formation of a granuloma surrounding an area of caseation leads to the appearance of primary lesion in the lung is known as Ghon's focus.

Q.148. What are the clinical features of pulmonary tuberculosis?

Ans. The clinical features of pulmonary tuberculosis are:

- Asymptomatic
- Symptomatic
  - Respiratory symptoms
    - Cough >3 weeks
    - Sputum production
    - Hemoptysis
    - Chest pain
    - Shortness of breath
    - Localized wheez.
  - General symptoms
    - Fever (low grade with evening rise of temperature and relieved at late night by sweating)
    - Weight loss
    - Anorexia.
- Signs
  - No physical signs in most of the cases
  - Signs of
    - Fibrosis
    - Collapse
    - Pleural effusion
    - Pneumothorax
    - Cavitary lesion may be found.

Q.149. What are the sites of extrapulmonary TB?

Ans. The sites of extrapulmonary TB are:

- Lymph node (20%–40%)—Cervical and supraclavicular are most common
- Serous membrane (like pleura 20%–25%, peritoneum)
- Meninges
- Intestine
- Genitourinary (5%–18%)
- Bones and joints
- Liver
- Adrenal gland.

Q.150. What are the organs resistant to develop TB?

Ans. The organs are:

- Cardiac muscle
- Skeletal muscle
- Thyroid gland
- Pancreas.

Q.151. What investigations are done to diagnose pulmonary TB?

Ans.
- Blood for
  - TC, DC, ESR, and Hb%
- CRP
- Radiology—
  - Chest X-ray
  - CT scan chest
- Bacteriological examination—Sputum for
  - Microscopic—ZN stain
  - Culture—Solid media (takes 4–6 weeks)
    - Lowenstein Jensen media
    - Middle Brook media
  - Liquid media (takes 1–3 weeks)
    - BACTEC media
    - MGIT (mycobacterial growth indicator tube) media
- Tuberculin skin test
  - Mantoux test
  - Heaf test
- Other—
  - PCR (10 colony is enough to become positive).

Q.152. What are the radiological presentations/findings of pulmonary tuberculosis?

Ans. The radiological presentations are:
- Soft patchy opacities
- Consolidation
- Collapse
- Cavitation
- Fibrosis
- Miliary shadowing
- Pleural effusion/empyema.

Q.153. What type of opacity is found in chest X-ray of a pulmonary TB patient?

Ans. Soft patchy opacities.

Q.154. What are the aims of treatment of tuberculosis?

Ans. The aims are:

- To interrupt TB transmission by rendering patient noninfectious thus reducing mortality and morbidity.
- To prevent development of drug resistance.

Q.155. What is the basis of combination therapy?

Ans. i. To prevent the emergence of resistance, e.g. INH acts on rapidly growing bacteria, pyrazinamide enters into the caseous material, refampicin acts on dormant bacilli.

ii. To prevent resistance due to spontaneous mutation.

Q.156. Why multidrug treatment is rational?

Ans. Multidrug treatment is rational due to:
- Better patient compliance
- Prevent drug resistance.

Q.157. What is FDC?

Ans. FDC means fixed dose combination, i.e. drugs are present in fixed amount in single tablet.

Q.158. What are the advantages of fixed drug combinations (FDC)?

Ans. The advantages of FDC are:
- Prescription errorless likely to occur due to straightforward dose recommendations and easier patient weight to dose adjustment.
- Small number of tablet to be ingested.
- Decreased drug resistance.

Q.159. Why long-term treatment is required?

Ans. Long-term treatment is required because:
- *Mycobacterium tuberculosis* multiplies slowly.
- Intensive phase rapidly reduces bacterial population.
- Continuation phase destroys the remaining bacteria.

Q.160. Define new case, relapse, treatment failure, treatment after default, and chronic TB?

Ans. **New case**—A patient who has never taken anti TB or taken for less than 1 month.

Relapse—A patient who recently received treatment and was cured or treatment completed and now again developed smear positive pulmonary TB.

Treatment failure—A patient while on management remain smear positive or becomes smear positive at 5 months or more after start of management or a patient who was initially smear negative and is found smear positive at the end of 2nd month of treatment.

Treatment after default—A patient who completed at least 1 month of treatment and returned after at least 2 months after interruption of treatment.

Chronic—A patient who remained smear positive after completing directly observed retreatment regimen.

Q.161. What are the drugs used in TB?

Ans. **1st line drugs**

- INH
- Rifampicin
- Pyrazinamide
- Ethambutol
- Streptomycin
- Thiacetazone.

2nd line drugs

- Aminoglycosides : Kanamycin and amikacin
- Thionamides: Ethionamide
- Fluoroquinolone
- Cycloserine
- Para-aminosalicylic acid
- Clofazimine and rifabutin.

Q.162. What is the treatment plan of TB according to national tuberculosis program (NTP)?

Ans. Treatment phase—

- **Initial or intensive phase**
- **Continuation phase**

Diagnostic category (adults)—

TB diagnostic category	Patient category	Treatment regimen	
		Intensive phase (Daily)	Continuation phase (Daily)
I	New smear (+) positive PTB patients New smear (–) negative PTB patients Extrapulmonary TB patients Concomitant associated HIV/AIDS	2(HRZE)	4(HR)

Contd...

Contd...

TB diagnostic category	Patient category	Treatment regimen	
		Intensive phase (Daily)	Continuation phase (Daily)
II	Sputum smear (+) positive PTB with of treatment of more than one month Relapse Treatment failure after Cat-I Treatment after default Others	2(HRZE)S/ 1(HRZE)	5(HR)E

Composition of FDC Tablets—

4FDC: Isoniazid 75 mg + rifampicin 150 mg + pyrazinamide 400 mg + ethambutol 275 mg

2FDC : Isoniazid 75 mg + rifampicin 150 mg

Dosages of FDC Tablets—

Category I:

Pretreatment weight (Kg)	Intensive phase Daily (First 2 months) Number of 4FDC tablets	Continuation phase Daily (Next 4 months) Number of 2FDC tablets
30–37	2	2
38–54	3	3
55–70	4	4
>70	5	5

Category II:

Pretreatment weight (Kg)	Intensive phase Daily (First 3 months)	Daily (First 2 months)	Continuation phase Daily (Next 5 months)	
	Number of 4FDC tablets	Injection streptomycin	Number of 2FDC tablets	Ethambutol 400 mg (Number of tablets)
30–37	2	500 mg	2	2

Contd...

Contd...

Pretreatment weight (Kg)	Intensive phase Daily (First 3 months)	Daily (First 2 months)	Continuation phase Daily (Next 5 months)	
	Number of 4FDC tablets	Injection streptomycin	Number of 2FDC tablets	Ethambutol 400 mg (Number of tablets)
38–54	3	700 mg	3	3
55–70	4	1 gm*	4	3
>70	5	1 gm*	5	4

NB: The dose of streptomycin should not exceed 750 mg daily after the age of 50 years.

Q.163. What is 6 months regimen?

Ans. Initial phase— 2 months.
Continuation phase—4 months.

Q.164. Name a single side effect from each of the 1st line anti-TB drugs?

Ans. Rifampicin — Hepatitis
INH—Peripheral neuropathy
Pyrazinamide—Hepatitis/ Hyperuricemia (gouty arthritis)
Ethambutol—Optic neuritis
Streptomycin—Ototoxicity (8th cranial nerve palsy)
Thiacetazone—Steven-Johnson's syndrome.

Q.165. A patient on anti-TB suddenly developed jaundice, how will you manage the patient?

Ans. Management of patient—

- Anti-TB drugs should be stopped.
- Liver function tests are done.
- Viral serology are done to exclude viral hepatitis.
- Supportive measures should be taken, e.g. nutrition.
- Wait till jaundice disappears and liver function returns to normal.
- After that anti-TB drugs will be reintroduced slowly.

Q.166. How will you investigate a case of sputum positive pulmonary TB?

Ans. After starting treatment with anti-TB drugs, sputum should be examined after 2, 3, and 5 months.

Q.167. How can you assess response to anti-TB treatment?

Ans. Treatment response—

- By 2nd week—Sputum smear becomes negative
- After 4 weeks—Feeling well, weight gain, no fever, no cough and sputum
- By 2 months—80% culture negative
- By 3 months—100% culture negative
- Chest radiograph— Should have improved.

Q.168. Why do we give BCG vaccine?

Ans. Causes of giving BCG vaccine are:

- Protection against tubercular meningitis and miliary tuberculosis.
- To protect the babies from TB which may be transmitted from mother or other source.
- Lack of maternal antibody against TB. The earlier the age, the higher the protection.

Q.169. How much protection can give BCG vaccine?

Ans. Protections are:

- BCG gives protection upto 7 years
- Protect in young 0%–70%.

Q.170. What are the types of drug resistant tuberculosis?

Ans. **Primary drug resistance**: It occurs in those exposed to others infected with resistant organism.

Secondary drug resistance: Occurs in patients who do not comply with the treatment regimen.

Multidrug resistance: Resistance to INH + rifampicin with or without other drug resistance.

XDRTB: Resistance to rifampicin +INH and any member of the quinolone and at least any of the injectable 2nd line drug.

Q.171. How do we prevent TB?

Ans. Prevention of TB:

- General health promotion
- Effective treatment of sputum positive case
- Specific protection

- Active immunization
- Chemoprophylaxis—INH 5 mg/kg/day for 9 months.

Q.172. What are the malignant conditions of lung?

Ans. The malignant conditions of lung are:

- Bronchogenic carcinoma
- Mesothelioma.

Q.173. What are the presentations of bronchogenic carcinoma?

Ans.
i. Asymptomatic—Detected as solitary nodule in X-ray.
ii. Local effects—Cough, hemoptysis, breathlessness, and collapse.
iii. Invasion of adjacent structures—Pleural pain, hoarseness of voice, and Horner's syndrome.
iv. Metastatic effects—Focal neurological deficit, epileptic seizures, personality change, jaundice, and bone pain or skin nodules.
v. Nonmetastatic extrapulmonary—SIADH, hypercalcemia, digital clubbing, etc.

Q.174. What are the causes of bronchogenic carcinoma?

Ans. Cigaret smoking — It is the most common cause of lung cancer. Radon and industrial materials (e.g. asbestos, silica, beryllium, cadmium, and chromium) are associated with lung cancer.

Q.175. What are the histological types of lung cancer?

Ans. Small-cell lung cancer— 20%

Nonsmall-cell lung cancer

- Squamous 35%
- Adenocarcinoma 30%

Large-cell 15%.

Q.176. What are nonmetastatic extrapulmonary manifestations of bronchial carcinoma?

Ans. **Endocrine—**

- Inappropriate antidiuretic hormone secretion causing hyponatremia.
- Ectopic adrenocorticotropic hormone secretion.
- Hypercalcemia due to secretion of parathyroid hormone-related peptides.
- Carcinoid syndrome.
- Gynecomastia.

Neurological—
- Polyneuropathy.
- Myelopathy.
- Cerebellar degeneration.
- Myasthenia (Lambert-Eaton syndrome).

Others—
- Digital clubbing.
- Hypertrophic pulmonary osteoarthropathy.
- Nephrotic syndrome.
- Polymyositis and dermatomyositis.
- Eosinophilia.

Q.177. What are the distant organs metastasized from bronchial carcinoma?

Ans. Distant metastases occur most commonly in bone, adrenals, liver, brain, and skin (BALBS).

Q.178. What investigations will you do for bronchial carcinoma?

Ans. The investigations are:
- Blood for TC, DC, Hb%, and ESR
- X-ray chest PA and lateral view
- Sputum for malignant cells
- Bronchoscopy and biopsy, bronchial brushing and washing
- CT scan and CT guided FNAC
- If palpable lymph node, biopsy
- If pleural effusion, pleural biopsy
- For metastases, USG of abdomen, CT scan of brain and abdomen, and isotope bone scan.

Q.179. What are the modalities of treatment?

Ans. The modalities of treatment are:
- Surgery
- Radiotherapy
- Chemotherapy
- Palliative therapy— Laser therapy and stenting, pain relieve.

Q.180. Which tumor is more sensitive to chemotherapy?

Ans. Small-cell carcinoma is more sensitive to chemotherapy.

Q.181. What are the primary sites of secondaries in the lung?

Ans. Breast, kidney, thyroid, ovary, uterus, and testes (BKTOUT).

Q.182. A young male presents with sudden severe right-sided chest pain and breathlessness. On examination, resonant on percussion and absent breath sound on right side. What is your diagnosis?

Ans. Right-sided pneumothorax is the diagnosis.

Q.183. What is pneumothorax?

Ans. Pneumothorax is the presence of air in the pleural space.

Q.184. What are the definitive signs of pneumothorax?

Ans. Hyper-resonant percussion note and diminished/absent breath sound.

Q.185. What are the causes of pneumothorax? Or classify pneumothorax.

Ans. Classification of pneumothorax

i. **Spontaneous**—
- Primary
  - No evidence of overt lung disease.
  - Rupture of—
    1. A small subpleural emphysematous bulla
    2. Pleural bleb
    3. The pulmonary end of a pleural adhesion.
- Secondary
  - Underlying lung disease, most commonly COPD and TB; asthma, lung abscess, pulmonary infarcts, and bronchogenic carcinoma.

ii. **Traumatic**—
- Iatrogenic (e.g. following thoracic surgery or biopsy, pleural fluid aspiration).
- Chest wall injury.

Q.186. What are the types of spontaneous pneumothorax?

Ans. The types of spontaneous pneumothorax are:
- Closed type.
- Open type.
- Tension (valvular) type.

Q.187. What are the features of tension pneumothorax?

Ans. The features of tension pneumothorax are:
- Severe chest pain
- Severe and progressive dyspnea
- Shifting of mediastinum
- Features of shock (cyanosis, hypotension, and tachycardia).

Q.188. What is the treatment of tension pneumothorax?

Ans. Immediate insertion of a needle in 2nd intercostal space in midclavicular line followed by water seal tube drainage.

Q.189. How can you treat pneumothorax?

Ans.
1. Tension pneumothorax, presence of chronic lung disease, age> 50 years with significant dyspnea/ occupying>15% of hemithorax, >2.5 L air aspiration—Water seal tube drainage.
2. Age< 50 years with significant dyspnea/occupying > 15% of hemithorax—Needle aspiration.
3. Insignificant dyspnea/occupying<15% of hemithorax—Observation.

Q.190. What are physical signs in bedside to differentiate lobar pneumonia and pneumothorax?

Ans.

Examination	Lobar pneumonia	Pneumothorax
Trachea	Central	Deviated to opposite site
Percussion note	Woody dull	Hyper-resonant
auscultation	Bronchial breath sound ↑ vocal resonance	↓ or absent breath sound ↓ or absent vocal resonance

CHAPTER 3

Gastrointestinal System

Q.1. What are the common presentations of gastrointestinal system?

Ans. Common symptoms of gastrointestinal disease are:

- Dysphagia and odynophagia
- Dyspepsia
- Vomiting
- Constipation
- Diarrhea
- Abdominal pain
- Weight loss
- Hematemesis
- Melena.

Q.2. Define dysphagia and odynophagia.

Ans. Dysphagia is defined as difficulty in swallowing. Odynophagia means painful swallowing.

Q.3. What are the types of dysphagia?

Ans. The types of dysphagia are:

- Oropharyngeal dysphagia
- Esophageal dysphagia.

Q.4. What are the causes of oropharyngeal dysphagia?

Ans. The causes of oropharyngeal dysphagia are:

- Bulbar palsy
- Pseudobulbar palsy
- Myasthenia gravis.

Q.5. What are the causes of esophageal dysphagia?

Ans. Stricture—

- Benign

- Peptic stricture
- Fibrous ring
- Malignant
  - Carcinoma of esophagus
  - Carcinoma of stomach
- Extrensic compression
- Esophagitis
  - Peptic esophagitis
  - Candidiasis
- Dysmotility–Achalasia.

Q.6. What are the differences between oropharyngeal and esophageal dysphagia?

Ans.

Oropharyngeal dysphagia	Esophageal dysphagia
Difficulty initiating swallowing +/– choking, nasal regurgitation or tracheal aspiration	Food 'sticking' after swallowing +/– regurgitation

Q.7. How will you investigate dysphagia?

Ans. The process of investigations are:

- Endoscopy of upper GI tract.
- Barium swallow with videofluoroscopic swallowing assessment.
- Esophageal manometry.

Q.8. What are the presentations of achalasia cardia?

Ans. The presentations of achalasia are:

i. The presentation is slowly developing dysphagia which is initially intermittent, and is worse for solids and eased by drinking liquids, and by standing and moving around after eating.
ii. Episodes of chest pain due to esophageal spasm.
iii. Nocturnal choking due to pulmonary aspiration.

Q.9. What is the management of achalasia cardia?

Ans. Management—

- Endoscopic—Pneumatic balloon dilatation using a 30–35 mm diameter.
- Surgical—Surgical myotomy (Heller's operation) with a partial fundoplication antireflux procedure.
- PPI therapy is often necessary after surgery.

Q.10. What is dyspepsia?

Ans. Dyspepsia is the medical term for indigestion, a

symptom that includes epigastric pain, heartburn, distension, nausea or 'an acid feeling' occurring after eating or drinking.

Q.11. What are the alarm features of dyspepsia?

Ans. Alarm features in dyspepsia are:

- Weight loss
- Anemia
- Vomiting
- Hematemesis and/or melena
- Dysphagia
- Palpable abdominal mass.

Q.12. What are the neurological causes of vomiting?

Ans. Neurological causes of vomiting are:

- Raised intracranial pressure, e.g. brain tumor
- Labyrinthitis and Meniere's disease
- Migraine
- Meningitis.

Q.13. Give the description of vomiting of gastric outlet obstruction, e.g. pyloric stenosis.

Ans. Projectile vomiting of large volumes of gastric content that is not bile-stained (green). Vomitus contains previous day food.

Q.14. Give the description of vomiting in raised intracranial pressure, e.g. brain tumor.

Ans. Vomiting is sudden, more in the morning without any warning, i.e. without nausea.

Q.15. What is hematemesis?

Ans. Hematemesis is the vomiting of blood.

Q.16. What is melena?

Ans. Melena is the passage of tarry black stool.

Q.17. How can you differentiate between hematemesis and hemoptysis?

Ans.

Hematemesis	Hemoptysis
Vomiting of blood	Coughing up blood
Coffee ground in color	Bright red in color
Mixed with food particle	Frothy, not mixed with food
Acidic reaction	Alkaline in reaction

Q.18. What are the common causes of hematemesis?

Ans. The common causes of hematemesis are:
- Peptic ulcer
- Gastric erosion
- Esophagitis
- Rupture esophageal varices
- Mallory–Weiss tear
- Carcinoma of stomach or esophagus
- Vascular malformation.

Q.19. What are the clinical features of upper GI bleeding?

Ans. Clinical features are:
- History of vomiting of blood or not.
- Features of shock—Pallor, cold extremities, thready pulse, and low blood pressure.
- Anemia—Iron deficiency anemia—Koloinychia, and pale smooth tongue.
- Stigmata of liver diseases such as jaundice, spider naevi, ascites, and splenomegaly.

Q.20. How much blood is lost to cause postural hypotension?

Ans. About 1.5 L blood is lost.

Q.21. How much blood is lost to produce shock?

Ans. About 3L blood is lost.

Q.22. What are the investigations done in acute upper GI bleeding?

Ans. Investigations are:
- Full blood count
- Blood grouping and crossmatching of at least 2 units of blood
- Urea and electrolytes
- Liver function test
- Prothrombin time
- Upper GI endoscopy.

Q.23. What is the management of acute upper GI bleeding?

Ans. Managements—
- Emergency management of acute nonvariceal upper gastrointestinal hemorrhage.
- Gain intravenous access with large-bore cannula.
- Check full blood count and routine biochemistry; crossmatch blood.

- Perform hourly measurements of blood pressure, pulse and urine output; consider central venous pressure (CVP) monitoring in severe bleeding.
- Give intravenous colloids or crystalloids in patients with hypotension and tachycardia.
- Transfuse with blood if blood pressure remains low and patient is actively bleeding.
- Organize endoscopy for diagnosis and treatment.
- Give IV PPI therapy for bleeding peptic ulcer.
- Consider surgery or arterial embolization if bleeding recurs.

Q.24. Which etiologies bear the worst prognosis?

Ans. Malignancy and varices have the worst prognosis.

Q.25. Mention the criteria of stool in melena?

Ans. Black, tarry, foul smelling, and sticky.

Q.26. How much blood is required to cause melena?

Ans. At least 60 mL blood in single episode is needed to cause melena.

Q.27. Why is stool black?

Ans. Stool is black due to formation of acid hematin as a result of lysis of RBC from upper GI bleeding.

Q.28. What are the usual sites for hematemesis and melena?

Ans. Upper gastrointestinal tract, especially stomach and duodenum are the usual sites but hemorrhage from upto the right side of the colon may cause melena.

Q.29. What are the causes of lower GI bleeding?

Ans. Causes of lower GI are:
- Anal disease, e.g. fissure, and hemorrhoids
- Inflammatory bowel disease
- Carcinoma
- Rectal polyps
- Angiodysplasia
- Solitary rectal ulcer
- Diverticular disease
- Meckel's diverticulum.

Q.30. Define diarrhea?

Ans. Passage of loose stool three or more times in a day is called diarrhea.

Or

Gastroenterologists define diarrhea as the passage of more than 200 gm of stool daily.

Diarrhea duration <2 weeks is called acute diarrhea and >2 weeks called chronic diarrhea.

Q.31. What are the causes of acute diarrhea?

Ans. Infective causes:

- Bacterial, e.g.
  - *Campylobacter jejuni*
  - Salmonella spp.
  - Shigella
  - *Escherichia coli*
  - Staphylococcal enterocolitis
  - *Bacillus cereus*
  - *Clostridium perfringens*, botulinum, and difficile
  - Gastrointestinal tuberculosis.
- Viral, e.g.
  - Rotavirus
- Fungal, e.g.
  - Histoplasmosis
- Parasitic, e.g.
  - Amebic dysentery (*Entamoeba histolytica*)
  - Giardia intestinalis

Noninfective causes of diarrhea:

- Drugs—Antibiotics, cytotoxic drugs, PPIs, and NSAIDs.

Q.32. What are the electrolyte imbalances occurring in acute watery diarrhea?

Ans. Electrolyte imbalances are:

- Hyponatremia
- Hypokalemia
- Metabolic acidosis, rarely alkalosis.

Q.33. What are the causes of bloody diarrhea?

Ans. Causes of bloody diarrhea are:

- Bacillary dysentery (Shigella)
- Amebic dysentery (*Entamoeba histolytica*)
- Inflammatory bowel disease
- Colonic carcinoma
- *Campylobacter jejuni*
- Salmonella spp.
- *Escherichia coli* (0157- H7)
- *Clostridium difficile*.

Q.34. Patient presented with acute watery diarrhea, how will you manage the patient?

Ans. Managements—

i. Assessment of dehydration

ii. Correction of dehydration according to degree of dehydration.
   - No dehydration—Liquid diet, increased amount of fluid intake
   - Some dehydration—By ORS (oral rehydration salt)
   - Severe dehydration—By IV fluid, e.g. cholera saline(100 mL/kg body wt. total, 40 mL/kg in first ½ hour and 60 mL/kg in next 2 and ½ hours in adult).

iii. If infective diarrhea, antimicrobials, e.g. azithromycin 1 gm or ciprofloxacin 1000 mg single dose in bacterial infection or nitazoxanide in rotavirus.

Q.35. What are the causes of chronic diarrhea?

Ans. The causes of chronic diarrhea are:

i. Irritable bowel syndrome
ii. Inflammatory bowel disease
iii. Colonic carcinoma
iv. Malabsorption—
   a. Pancreatic—
      - Chronic pancreatitis
      - Cancer of pancreas
   b. Enteropathy—
      - Celiac disease
      - Tropical sprue
      - Lymphoma
      - Lymphangiectasia
   c. Small bowel—
      - Gastrointestinal tuberculosis
      - Drugs— NSAIDs
      - VIPoma.

Q.36. What is the most common cause of chronic diarrhea?

Ans. Irritable bowel syndrome (IBS) is the most common cause of chronic diarrhea.

Q.37. What is steatorrhea?

Ans. Steatorrhea is fatty stools, pale, bulky, greasy, and difficult to flush.

Q.38. What are the mechanisms responsible for malabsorption?

Ans. Mechanisms are:
- Intraluminal maldigestion
- Mucosal malabsorption
- 'Postmucosal' lymphatic obstruction.

Q.39. Define constipation.

Ans. Constipation is defined as infrequent passage of hard stools.

Q.40. What is the most common cause of constipation?

Ans. Simple idiopathic constipation is the most common cause of constipation.

Q.41. What are the neurological causes of constipation?

Ans. Neurological causes of constipation are:

- Multiple sclerosis
- Spinal cord lesions
- Cerebrovascular accidents
- Parkinsonism.

Q.42. What are the metabolic/endocrine causes of constipation?

Ans. Metabolic endocrine causes of constipation are:

- Diabetes mellitus (autonomic neuropathy)
- Hypercalcemia
- Hypothyroidism
- Pregnancy.

Q.43. What are the types of laxative?

Ans. Types of laxative—

i. Bulk-forming laxatives
   - Dietary fiber
   - Wheat bran
   - Methylcellulose
   - Mucilaginous seeds and seed coats, e.g. ispaghula husk.

ii. Stimulant laxatives (stimulate motility and intestinal secretion)
   - Bisacodyl
   - Anthraquinones—Senna and dantron
   - Docusate sodium.

iii. Osmotic laxatives
   - Magnesium sulfate
   - Lactulose.

Q.44. Tell five common causes of pathological weight loss.

Ans. Five common causes of pathological weight loss are:

- Diabetes mellitus
- Tuberculosis
- Thyrotoxicosis
- Malignancy
- Malabsorption/malnutrition.

Q.45. What do you mean by significant weight loss?

Ans. More than 3 kg loss in 6 months or 10% of body weight in 6 month or 0.5 kg/month.

Q.46. What are the causes of weight loss with increased appetite?

Ans. Causes of weight loss with increased appetite are:
- Diabetes mellitus
- Thyrotoxicosis.

Q.47. What are the causes of acute abdominal pain (acute abdomen)?

Ans. Causes of acute abdominal pain are:

i. Inflammation
  - Appendicitis
  - Diverticulitis
  - Cholecystitis
  - Pelvic inflammatory disease
  - Pancreatitis
  - Pyelonephritis
  - Intra-abdominal abscess.

ii. Perforation/rupture
  - Peptic ulcer
  - Diverticular disease
  - Ovarian cyst
  - Aortic aneurysm.

iii. Obstruction
  - Intestinal obstruction
  - Biliary colic
  - Ureteric colic.

Q.48. What are the medical causes of acute abdominal pain (acute abdomen)?

Ans. Medical causes of acute abdominal pain are:
- Peptic ulcer
- Pancreatitis
- Pyelonephritis
- Diabetic ketoacidosis
- Addison's disease
- Acute intermittent porphyria
- Hypercalcemia.

Q.49. What are the causes of abdominal distension?

Ans. Causes of abdominal distension are:
- 5Fs

- Fat
- Fluid (ascites)
- Feces
- Flatus
- Fetus.

Q.50. Define GERD.

Ans. GERD develops when the esophageal mucosa is exposed to gastroduodenal contents for prolong period of time, resulting in symptoms and, in a proportion of cases, esophagitis.

Q.51. What are the clinical features of GERD?

Ans. Clinical features of GERD—

- Heartburn and regurgitation provoked by bending, straining or lying down.
- Waterbrush-salivation due to reflex salivary gland stimulation.
- Odynophagia or dysphagia—Woken at night by choking as refluxed fluid irritates the larynx.
- Atypical chest pain (can mimic angina).

Q.52. What are the complications of GERD?

Ans. Complication of GERD are:

- Esophagitis
- Barrett's esophagus
- Anemia (iron deficiency anemia)
- Benign esophageal stricture (as a consequence of long-standing esophagitis).

Q.53. How can you treat GERD?

Ans. Treatment of GERD—

1. Lifestyle advice:
   - Elevation of bed head in those who experience nocturnal symptoms
   - Avoidance of dietary items which the patient finds worsen symptoms
   - Avoidance of late meals
   - Weight reduction
   - Giving up smoking.
2. Antacids and alginates provide symptomatic benefit
3. H2 receptor antagonist
4. PPI is the treatment of choice
5. Laparoscopic antireflux surgery.

Q.54. What is Barrett's esophagus?

Ans. Barrett's esophagus is a premalignant condition in which the normal squamous lining of the lower esophagus is replaced by columnar mucosa (columnar lined esophagus; CLO) containing areas of intestinal metaplasia.

Q.55. What is PUD?

Ans. The term 'peptic ulcer' refers to an ulcer in the lower esophagus, stomach or duodenum, in the jejunum after surgical anastomosis to the stomach or, rarely, in the ileum adjacent to a Meckel's diverticulum.

Q.56. What are the common sites of PUD?

Ans. The common sites of PUD are:

i. Stomach
ii. Duodenum
iii. Lower end of esophagus
iv. In the jejunum after surgical anastomosis to the stomach
v. In the ileum adjacent to a Meckel's diverticulum.

Q.57. Is PUD possible in ileum?

Ans. Yes, adjacent to a Meckel's diverticulum.

Q.58. What are the causes of peptic ulcer disease (PUD)?

Ans. Causes of peptic ulcer disease are:

i. *Helicobacter pylori*: Peptic ulceration is strongly associated with *H.pylori* infection. Around 90% of duodenal ulcer patients and 70% of gastric ulcer patients are infected with *H. pylori*.
ii. *NSAID*: Damage mucosal barrier, reduce integrity of the duodenal mucosa, and increase the risk of bleeding or perforation from pre-existing gastric/duodenal ulcer.
iii. *Stress ulcer*: Curling and Cushing's ulcer.
iv. Zollinger-Ellison syndrome.
v. *Smoking*: Increases risk of gastric ulcer and to lesser extent duodenal ulcer.
vi. Blood group A.

Q.59. Which NSAIDs has very low risk in PUD?

Ans. NSAIDs with very low risk in PUD is:

- Celecoxib
- Etoricoxib.

Q.60. What are the consequences of *H. pylori* infection?

Ans. Consequences of *H. pylori* infection are:
- Chronic gastritis
- Peptic ulcer disease
- Gastric carcinoma
- MALToma (mucosa associated lymphoid tissue).

Q.61. What are the characteristics of peptic ulcer pain?

Ans. Characteristics of peptic ulcer are:
- It is episodic in nature
- Localization to epigastrium
- Nocturnal
- Pointing sign positive
- Relationship to food.

Q.62. How can you investigate PUD?

Ans. Investigations of PUD—

i. Upper GI endoscopy (confirmatory)

ii. Test for detection of *H.pylori* infection

  a. Invasive (endoscopy/biopsy required)
    - Rapid urease test
    - Histology
    - Culture

  b. Noninvasive
    - Serology
    - Urea breath test
    - Stool antigen

iii. Barium meal X-ray of stomach and duodenum(less used nowadays).

Q.63. What are the diagnostic and prognostic values of endoscopy?

Ans. Diagnostic and prognostic values of endoscopy are:
- Endoscopy is the confirmatory diagnostic tool for PUD (92% sensitive but 100% specific). It can exclude other lesions.
- Endoscopy can be used to see whether ulcer heals or not.

Q.64. What are the complications of PUD?

Ans. Complications of PUD are:
- GI bleeding
- Perforation
- Gastric outlet obstruction.

Q.65. What are the endoscopic criteria of rebleeding?

Ans. Endoscopic criteria of rebleeding are:

- Ulcer with active bleeding — Oozing and sprouting
- Ulcer with adjacent clot
- Ulcer with visible blood vessel on the base.

Q.66. How can you treat PUD?

Ans. Treatment of PUD:

i. *H.pylori* eradication:
   A. 1st line therapy (triple therapy) for 7 days
   - PPI 12-hourly
   - Clarithromycin 500 mg 12-hourly
   - Amoxicillin 1 gm 12-hourly or metronidazole 400 mg 12-hourly. If fails then

   B. 2nd line therapy for 7 days
   - PPI 12-hourly
   - Bismuth 120 mg 6-hourly
   - Metronidazole 400 mg 12-hourly
   - Tetracycline 500 mg 6-hourly.

ii. General measures: Smoking, aspirin and NSAIDs should be avoided

iii. Maintenance treatment: PPI should be used for 6–8 weeks.

iv. Surgical treatment
   Superselective vagotomy.

Q.67. What is the management of endoscopically found PUD?

Ans. Managements are:

- *H.pylori* status should be assessed.
- If *H.pylori* is positive, triple therapy.
- If *H.pylori* is negative, PPI.

Q.68. What is triple therapy?

Ans. Triple therapy is a regimen containing three drugs including a PPI taken simultaneously with two antibiotics from amoxicillin, clarithromycin and metronidazole.

Q.69. What are the indications for *H. pylori* eradication?

Ans. Indications are—

- Peptic ulcer
- MALToma
- *H. pylori*—Positive dyspepsia.

Q.70. What are the indications for surgery in peptic ulcer?

Ans. i. Emergency
- Perforation
- Hemorrhage

ii. Elective
- Complications, e.g. gastric outflow obstruction
- Recurrent ulcer following gastric surgery.

Q.71. What are the complications after PUD surgery?

Ans. Complications after PUD surgery are:
- Dumping
- Bile reflux gastritis
- Diarrhea and maldigestion
- Weight loss
- Anemia
- Metabolic bone disease
- Gastric cancer.

Q.72. What is dumping syndrome?

Ans. Dumping is a complication of gastric surgery. Rapid gastric emptying leads to distension of the proximal small intestine as the hypertonic contents draw fluid into the lumen. This leads to abdominal discomfort and diarrhea after eating. Autonomic reflexes release a range of gastrointestinal hormones which lead to vasomotor features such as flushing, palpitations, sweating, tachycardia and hypotension.

Q.73. What are the common presentations of carcinoma of stomach?

Ans. Common presentations of carcinoma of stomach are:
- Patients above 40 years may present with 3As—Anemia, anorexia and asthenia
- Epigastric pain—Epigastric, severe, partly meal related, not relieved by antacid
- Epigastric mass
- Vomiting (if it is in pylorus)
- Dysphagia (if it is in cardiac end)
- Dyspepsia, hematemesis and melena
- Unexplained iron-deficiency anemia
- Features of metastasis.

Q.74. What are the paraneoplastic features of carcinoma of the stomach?

Ans. Paraneoplastic features of carcinoma of the stomach are:
- *Acanthosis nigricans*
- Thrombophlebitis (Trousseau's sign)
- Dermatomyositis.

Q.75. Tell the sites of carcinoma of the stomach.

Ans. Sites of carcinoma of the stomach are:
- Antrum—50%
- Cardiac end—20%
- Body of the stomach—20%–30%.

Q.76. How can you confirm the diagnosis?

Ans. Endoscopy of upper GI tract and biopsy.

Q.77. What are the modalities of treatment?

Ans. Modalities of treatment are:
- Surgery
- Chemotherapy
- Palliative therapy.

Q.78. Describe the pain of acute pancreatitis.

Ans. Severe, constant upper abdominal pain which radiates to the back builds up over 15–60 minutes immediately after eating, relieved by stupping forward.

Q.79. What are the characteristic findings on examination?

Ans. Characteristic findings on examination are:
- Marked epigastric tenderness in spite of little guarding and rigidity.
- Discoloration of the flanks (Grey Turner's sign) or the periumbilical region (Cullen's sign)—Features of severe pancreatitis with hemorrhage.

Q.80. Mention the common causes of acute pancreatitis?

Ans. Common causes of acute pancreatitis are—
- Gallstones
- Alcohol
- Idiopathic
- Post-ERCP
- Infection (mumps and coxsackievirus)
- Metabolic (hypercalcemia and hypertriglyceridemia)

- Drugs (azathioprine, thiazide, diuretics, sodium valproate).

Q.81. What are the adverse prognostic factors in acute pancreatitis (Glasgow criteria)?

Ans. Adverse prognostic factors are:

- Age > 55 years
- PO_2 < 8 kPa (60 mmHg)
- White blood cell count (WBC) > 15 × 10^9/L
- Albumin < 32 gm/L
- Serum calcium < 2 mmol/L (8 mg/dL) (corrected)
- Glucose > 10 mmol/L (180 mg/dL)
- Urea > 16 mmol/L (45 mg/dL) (after rehydration)
- Alanine aminotransferase (ALT) > 200 U/L
- Lactate dehydrogenase (LDH) > 600 U/L.

Q.82. How can you investigate acute pancreatitis?

Ans. Investigations in acute pancreatitis are:

- S. amylase (after 24 hours urinary amylase)
- S. lipase
- USG of hepatobiliary system including pancreas (pancreatic swelling, gallstone)
- Plain X-ray of abdomen to exclude other pathology
- Blood urea and S.electrolytes
- Blood glucose
- S.ALT, LDH
- S.calcium and WBC count.

Q.83. What are the causes of raised serum amylase other than acute pancreatitis?

Ans. Causes of raised serum amylase other than acute pancreatitis are:

- Upper gastrointestinal perforation
- Biliary peritonitis
- Intestinal infarction
- Macroamylasemia.

Q.84. What is the role of serum lipase in diagnosis of acute pancreatitis?

Ans. Serum lipase is raised in acute pancreatitis and this remains elevated for a longer period of time than those of amylase but the accuracy of serum lipase is not significantly greater than serum amylase and it is technically more difficult to measure.

Q.85. Write down the treatment of acute pancreatitis?

Ans. Treatment of acute pancreatitis are:
- NPO
- Analgesic: Pethidine with atropine (relax sphincter of Oddi), tramadol
- IV fluids—Normal saline/colloids to correct hypovolemia.
- Hyperglycemia is corrected by insulin
- Prophylactic broad spectrum intravenous antibiotics such as imipenem or cefuroxime in severe cases
- Treatment of the cause.

Q.86. What are the complications of acute pancreatitis?

Ans. Complications are—

i. Systemic
   - Hyperglycemia
   - Hypocalcemia
   - Hypoxia

ii. Pancreatic
   - Abscess
   - Pseudocyst
   - Pancreatic ascites or pleural effusion

iii. Gastrointestinal
   - Upper gastrointestinal bleeding
   - Duodenal obstruction
   - Obstructive jaundice.

Q.87. What is the most common cause of chronic pancreatitis?

Ans. Alcohol is the most common cause of chronic pancreatitis.

Q.88. What are the causes of chronic/recurrent pancreatitis?

Ans. Causes of chronic/recurrent pancreatitis are:
- Alcohol
- Tropical chronic pancreatitis
- Hereditary chronic pancreatitis
- Cystic fibrosis
- Idiopathic chronic pancreatitis
- Trauma
- Hypercalcemia.

Q.89. What are the cardinal features of chronic pancreatitis?

Ans. Cardinal features of chronic pancreatitis are:

- Recurrent abdominal pain
- Chronic diarrhea and steatorrhea
- Diabetes mellitus
- Weight loss.

Q.90. What is IBS?

Ans. Irritable bowel syndrome (IBS) is a functional bowel disorder characterized by altered bowel habits, abdominal pain, and absence of detectable organic pathology. IBS is the most common GI disease in clinical practice.

Q.91. What are the types/clinical presentations of IBS?

Ans. Three types/clinical presentations:

1. Spastic colon (constipation predominant)
2. Alternating constipation and diarrhea (mixed)
3. Chronic painless diarrhea (diarrhea predominant).

Q.92. What are the diagnostic criteria of IBS?

Ans. Recurrent abdominal pain or discomfort at least 3 days/month in the last 3 months associated with two or more of the followings:

1. Improvement with defecation
2. Onset associated with a change in frequency of stool
3. Onset associated with a change in form (appearance) of stool.

Q.93. What are the clinical features of IBS?

Ans. Clinical features of IBS are:

- Colicky abdominal pain
- Altered bowel habit
- Abdominal distension
- Rectal mucus
- Feeling of incomplete defecation.

Q.94. What are the characteristics of pain in IBS?

Ans. Recurrent abdominal pain which is usually colicky or 'cramping' in nature, felt in the lower abdomen and relieved by defecation.

Q.95. What are the negative criteria of IBS?

Ans. Negative criteria of IBS—

- Age > 40 years
- Weight loss
- Nocturnal symptoms
- Blood in stool.

Q.96. Write down the difference between IBS and IBD.

Ans.

Traits	IBS	IBD
Types of disease	Functional bowel disorder	Inflammatory
Ulcer in the GIT	No	Yes
Predominant clinical features	Altered bowel habit and abdominal pain	Blood diarrhea
Complications	Less	More
Treatment	Reassurance, medical and psychotherapy	Prompt medical and surgical treatment

Q.97. What is the treatment of diarrhea predominant IBS?

Ans. Treatment of diarrhea predominant IBS are:

- Reassurance
- Avoid excessive dietary fiber and legume
- Antidiarrheal drugs—Loparamide, codeine phosphate
- Amitriptyline
- Hypnotherapy.

Q.98. What is the treatment of constipation predominant IBS?

Ans. Treatment of constipation predominant IBS are:

- Reassurance
- High roughage diet
- Ispaghula, lactulose
- Relaxation therapy.

Q.99. What do you mean by IBD?

Ans. IBD means inflammatory bowel disease.

Q.100. Which diseases are included under IBD?

Ans. Ulcerative colitis and Crohn's disease are included under IBD.

Q.101. Where is the site of lesion in ulcerative colitis?

Ans. Colon only; begins at anorectal margin with variable proximal extension.

Q.102. Where is the site of lesion in Crohn's disease?

Ans. Any part of gastrointestinal tract from mouth to anus. The sites most commonly involved, in order of frequency, are terminal ileum and right side of colon, colon alone, terminal ileum alone, ileum and jejunum.

Q.103. What are the characteristics of lesions in ulcerative colitis?

Ans. Characteristics of lesions in ulcerative colitis are continuous mucosal and submucosal inflammation.

Q.104. What are the characteristics of lesions in Crohn's disease?

Ans. Characteristics of lesions in Crohn's disease are noncontinuous or discrete transmural inflammation.

Q.105. What is the most common presentation of ulcerative colitis?

Ans. Bloody diarrhea is the most common presentation of ulcerative colitis.

Q.106. What are the complications of inflammatory bowel disease?

Ans. Complications of inflammatory bowel disease are:

- Intestinal
  - Life-threatening colonic inflammation (toxic megacolon)
  - Hemorrhage
  - Fistulas
  - Cancer
- Extraintestinal—
  - Eyes
    - Uveitis
    - Episcleritis
    - Conjunctivitis
  - Joints
    - Type I (pauciarticular) arthropathy
    - Type II (polyarticular) arthropathy
    - Arthralgia
    - Ankylosing spondylitis
    - Inflammatory back pain
  - Skin
    - Erythema nodosum
    - Pyoderma gangrenosum
  - Liver and biliary tree
    - Sclerozing cholangitis
    - Fatty liver
    - Chronic hepatitis
    - Cirrhosis
    - Gallstones
  - Nephrolithiasis
    - Stones in patients with small bowel disease or after resection.
- Venous thrombosis.

Q.107. What extraintestinal features are associated with active disease of IBD?

Ans. Eyes
- Uveitis
- Episcleritis
- Conjunctivitis

Joints
- Arthralgia of large joints

Skin
- Erythema nodosum
- Pyoderma gangrenosum
- Mouth ulcer

Liver and biliary tree
- Sclerozing cholangitis
- Fatty liver
- Chronic hepatitis
- Cirrhosis
- Gallstones
- Venous thrombosis.

Q.108. How can you differentiate ulcerative colitis from Crohn's disease?

Ans.

	Ulcerative colitis	Crohn's disease
Risk factors	More common in non/ exsmokers	More common in smokers
Anatomical distribution	Colon only; begins at anorectal margin with variable proximal extension	Any part of gastrointestinal tract; perianal disease common; patchy distribution —'skip lesions'
Presentation	Bloody diarrhea	Variable; pain, diarrhea, weight loss all common
Histology	Inflammation limited to mucosa; crypt distortion, cryptitis, crypt abscesses, loss of goblet cells	Submucosal or transmural inflammation common; deep fissuring ulcers, fistulas; patchy changes; granulomas
Management	5-ASA; corticosteroids; azathioprine; colectomy is curative	Corticosteroids; azathioprine; methotrexate; biologic therapy (anti-TNF); nutritional therapy; surgery for complications is not curative

Q.109. What are the drugs used in the treatment of IBD?

Ans. Drugs used in the treatment of IBD are:

- Aminosalicylates (mesalazine, olsalazine, sulfasalazine, balsalazide)
- Corticosteroids (prednisolone, hydrocortisone, budesonide)
- Azathioprine
- Methotrexate
- Anti-TNF antibodies (infliximab and adalimumab).

Q.110. What are the features of severe ulcerative colitis?

Ans. Features of severe ulcerative colitis are:

- Stool frequency> 6 stools/day
- Blood in stool +++
- Fever >37.5°C, 2 days out of 4
- Tachycardia >90/minute
- ESR> 30 mm/hour
- Anemia< 10 gm/dL Hb
- Albumin <30 gm/L.

Q.111. How can you manage severe/fulminant ulcerative colitis?

Ans. Medical management of fulminant ulcerative colitis are:

- Intravenous fluids.
- Transfusion if Hb < 100 gm/L.
- IV methylprednisolone (60 mg daily) or hydrocortisone (400 mg daily).
- Antibiotics for proven infection.
- Nutritional support.
- Subcutaneous heparin for prophylaxis of venous thromboembolism.
- Avoidance of opiates and antidiarrheal agents.
- Consider infliximab (5 mg/kg) in stable patients not responding to 3–5 days of corticosteroids.

Q.112. Name some diseases which affect the terminal ileum?

Ans. Diseases which affect the terminal ileum are followings:

- Intestinal tuberculosis
- Crohn's disease
- Lymphoma
- *Yersinia enterocolitica.*

Q.113. What are the presentations of intestinal TB?

Ans. Presentations of intestinal TB are:

- Abdominal pain—Acute or chronic
- Alteration of bowel habit—Diarrhea alternating with constipation
- Low-grade fever
- Abdominal swelling due to ascites in peritoneal tuberculosis.

Q.114. What are the pathological types of intestinal TB?

Ans. Pathological types of intestinal TB are:

- Ulcerative
- Hypertrophic
- Mixed.

Q.115. What are the indications of steroid in TB?

Ans. Indications of steroid in TB are:

- Tubercular meningitis
- Miliary tuberculosis
- Tubercular pericarditis
- Urogenital tuberculosis.

Q.116. What are the causes of oral ulcer?

Ans. Causes of oral ulceration are:

- Aphthous
- Infection
  - Candidiasis
  - Herpes simplex
  - Syphilis.
- Gastrointestinal diseases
  - Crohn's disease
  - Celiac disease.
- Dermatological conditions
  - Lichen planus
  - Pemphigoid
  - Pemphigus
  - Stevens-Johnson syndrome.
- Cytotoxic drugs
- Systemic diseases
  - Systemic lupus erythematosus (SLE)

  - Behçet's syndrome.
- Neoplasia
  - Carcinoma
  - Leukemia
  - Kaposi's sarcoma.

Q.117. What are aphthous ulcers?

Ans. Aphthous ulcers are superficial and painful oral ulcer either idiopathic or premenstrual.

CHAPTER 4

Hepatology

Q.1. What is jaundice?

Ans. Jaundice is the yellowish coloration of skin, sclera and mucous membrane due to raised level of bilirubin in the plasma.

Q.2. At which level of bilirubin jaundice is clinically detected?

Ans. Jaundice is usually detectable clinically when the plasma bilirubin exceeds 50 µmol/L (3 mg/dL).

Q.3. What are the types of jaundice?

Ans. Types of jaundice are:

Prehepatic—Hemolytic or congenital hyperbilirubinemia

Hepatic—Hepatocellular jaundice

Posthepatic—Obstructive (cholestatic) jaundice.

Q.4. Define hepatitis.

Ans. Necroinflammation of hepatic parenchyma is called hepatitis.

Q.5. What are the common causes of hepatitis?

Ans. Common causes of hepatitis are:

- Viral hepatitis
- Drugs
- Alcohol
- Autoimmune.

Q.6. Name the drugs causing hepatitis.

Ans. Drugs are:

- Pyrazinamide

- Halothane
- Isoniazid
- Rifampicin
- Allopurinol
- Amitriptylin
- Azathioprin
- Indomethacin
- Ibuprofen
- Amiodarone.

Q.7. What are the causes of viral hepatitis?

Ans. Causes of viral hepatitis are:

Common—Hepatitis virus
- Hepatitis A
- Hepatitis B ± hepatitis D
- Hepatitis C
- Hepatitis E

Less common—Other viruses
- Cytomegalovirus
- Epstein-Barr virus
- Herpes simplex
- Yellow fever.

Q.8. What are the hepatotropic viruses?

Ans. Hepatotropic viruses are:
- Hepatitis A
- Hepatitis B ± hepatitis D
- Hepatitis C
- Hepatitis E
- Cytomegalovirus
- Epstein-Barr virus.

Q.9. Classify viral hepatitis.

Ans. i. Etiological classification:

a. Major hepatotropic viruses:
   - HAV
   - HBV
   - HCV
   - HDV
   - HEV.

b. Minor hepatotropic virus:
   - HGV

c. Transfusion transmitted virus (TTV)
d. Tropical virus:
- Yellow fever virus
- Dengue flavivirus
- Hemorrhagic virus
e. Systemic virus:
- Herpes virus
- EBV
- CMV.

ii. Clinical classification:
- Acute (inflammation less than 6 months)
- Chronic (inflammation more than 6 months).

Q.10. Which hepatitis viruses cause acute viral hepatitis?

Ans. Hepatitis viruses cause acute viral hepatitis are:
- Hepatitis A
- Hepatitis B ± hepatitis D
- Hepatitis E.

Q.11. Which hepatitis viruses cause chronicity?

Ans. Hepatitis viruses cause chronicity are:
- Hepatitis B ± hepatitis D
- Hepatitis C.

Q.12. What are the genomic types of hepatitis viruses?

Ans. All are RNA viruses except HBV which is DNA virus.

Q.13. Can HDV itself cause disease?

Ans. No, as HDV is a defective virus it works along with HBV.

Q.14. What is the mode of transmission of each virus?

Ans. a. Hepatitis A and Hepatitis E – Feco-oral route

b. Hepatitis B ± hepatitis D—
i. Horizontal transmission
- Infected unscreened blood products
- IV drug use
- Tattoos/acupuncture needles
- Sexual (homosexual and heterosexual)
- Surgical procedure

ii. Vertical transmission

c. Hepatitis C—
- Parenteral transmission
- Infected unscreened blood products
- IV drug use
- Tattoos/acupuncture needles.

Q.15. What is feco-oral route?

Ans. When organism enters through mouth by ingestion of contaminated food or drinks.

Q.16. What is the classical patterns of acute viral hepatitis?

Ans. Classical patterns are:

i. Prodromal phase: Usually 2 weeks, influenza like symptoms. Nausea, vomiting, distaste for cigaret, constant right upper abdominal pain (due to stretching of Glisson's capsule).

ii. Icteric phase: Jaundice, liver is palpable, soft and tender. Spleen is palpable in 10% cases particularly in children, appetite returns to normal.

iii. Recovery phase: Uninterrupted (once in recovery phase patient become well spontaneously), duration of recovery within 6 months (usually 2–4 weeks).

Q.17. What investigations can be done in acute viral hepatits?

Ans. Investigations are:

i. LFT (liver function test)
- Serum bilirubin (to see depth of jaundice)
- SGPT (ALT)— Increase (release from damaged hepatocytes)
- Serum ALP (increase in biliary intrahepatic obstruction)
  - ALT>6 times, ALP<2.5 times is suggestive of hepatocellular jaundice, ALT<6 times and ALP>2.5 times is in favor of cholestatic jaundice.
- PT—Increase (most important prognostic factor)
- Serum albumin (if jaundice > 25 days albumin decrease since half-life of albumin 25 days)

ii. Serology
- Hepatitis A: Anti-HAV IgM (Acute infection)
- Hepatitis B: HBsAg, anti-HBc IgM, HBeAg,
- Hepatitis C: Anti-HCV antibody, HCV-RNA.
- Hepatitis E: Anti-HEV IgM,

iii. USG—Hepatomegaly, uniform hypoechoic echotexture

iv. CBC—ESR increase, relative lymphocytosis.

Q.18. Can you tell significance of antigen and antibody of HBV?

Ans. Significance are:

i. HBsAg—It indicates infection with HBV (acute and chronic). HBsAg appears in the blood late in the incubation period but before the prodromal phase of acute type B hepatitis; it usually lasts for 3–4 weeks and can persist for upto 5 months.

ii. HBsAb— It appears 3 months after onset and persist. It indicates either a previous infection, in which case anti-HBc is usually also present or previous vaccination, in which case anti-HBc is not present.
iii. HBeAg— It indicates viral replication.
iv. HBeAb— It indicates low infectivity
v. HBcAb IgM—Acute hepatitis B
vi. HBcAb IgG — Previous or chronic infection.

Q.19. What are the components of liver function tests?

Ans. Components of LFTs are:
- Serum bilirubin
- Aminotransferase (ALT and AST)
- Alkaline phosphatase
- Gamma-glutamyl transferase
- Serum albumin
- Prothrombin time.

Q.20. What is window period? Which marker will be found in this period?

Ans. Window period is the period between disappearance of HBsAg and appearance of anti-HBs.

During this period anti-HBc IgM is always positive.

Q.21. What are the complications of acute viral hepatitis?

Ans. Complications of acute viral hepatitis are:
- Acute liver failure
- Relapsing hepatitis
- Cholestatic hepatitis (hepatitis A)
- Aplastic anemia
- Chronic liver disease and cirrhosis (hepatitis B and C).

Q.22. How can you treat acute viral hepatitis?

Ans. i. Treatment of acute attack:
- Rest
- Diet—No specific dietary modifications are needed. Avoid drugs such as sedatives and narcotics, which are metabolized in the liver, alcohol, elective surgery.

ii. Treatment of complications—Liver transplantation in acute liver failure if it develops.
iii. Follow-up— LFT (Serum bilirubin, ALT, PT)

- 3–4 weeks after discharge, monthly for next 3 months.
- Special attention— Recurrence of jaundice.

iv. Prevention—
- Improvement of sanitation
- Vaccination.

Q.23. What is the indication of hospital admission?

Ans. Severe anorexia/vomiting/electrolyte imbalance requiring IV fluid and nutrition biochemical changes like—
- Rising serum bilirubin > 15 mg/dL
- Rising of PT
- Rapid falling of aminotransferase level despite rising bilirubin
- Persistence of hyperbilirubinemia at plateau for 2–3 weeks.

Encephalopathy (hepatic failure)—Change of mentation, flapping tremor.

Q.24. A 15-year-old boy is diagnosed, he is suffering from acute viral hepatitis but HBsAg is negative. Which virus will you think next?

Ans. Hepatitis A virus.

Q.25. Why?

Ans. It is more common in developing countries and spread by feco-oral route.

Q.26. What is the prognosis of acute hepatitis due to hepatitis A?

Ans. Prognosis is good. Acute liver failure is rare in hepatitis A (0.1%) and chronic infection does not occur.

Q.27. A 35-year-old lady is diagnosed, he is suffering from acute viral hepatitis but HBsAg is negative. Which virus will you think next?

Ans. Hepatitis E virus.

Q.28. Why?

Ans. In developing countries, by this age person becomes immune to hepatitis A due to clinical or subclinical infection.

Q.29. Suppose this lady is pregnant, what is your concern?

Ans. Special care should be given as there is increased chance of developing acute liver failure and mortality rate is 20% in pregnant women with HEV infection.

Q.30. What are the fates of hepatitis B virus infection?

Ans. The fates of hepatitis B virus infection are:

i. Asymptomatic
ii. Acute hepatitis (90%):
- Recovery—99%
- Acute liver failure and death rate is 1%

iii. Chronicity (10%)— HBsAg +ve for >6 months
- Resolution
- Asymptomatic
- Carrier state
- Chronic persistent hepatitis
- Chronic active hepatitis
  - Extrahepatic complications: PAN, GN
  - Cirrhosis
  - HCC – Death.

Q.31. How many patients with hepatitis B virus infection develop chronicity?

Ans. It depends on route of transmission—
- Horizontal transmission (10%)
- Vertical transmission (90%).

Q.32. What are the drugs used to treat chronic hepatitis B?

Ans. Drugs are:
- Interferon-alfa
- Lamivudine
- Adefovir
- Entecavir and telbivudine
- Tenofovir.

Q.33. Tell the indications of antiviral therapy.

Ans. Indications are:

i. HBeAg positive patients—
   HBV DNA>20000 IU/mL with serum ALT>2 times normal, should be treated.
   Liver biopsy is not essential in this group.
   HBV DNA levels >20000 IU/L with serum ALT <2 times normal, should not be treated.
   A liver biopsy may help as treatment is sometimes given if inflammation is marked.

ii. HBeAg negative patients—
   HBV DNA >20000 IU should also be treated if ALT>2 times.

HBV DNA >2000 IU should have a liver biopsy to help with the decision to treat or not.

iii. Compensated cirrhosis patients—
HBV DNA>2000 IU/L should be treated.
HBV DNA <2000 should only be treated if the ALT is high.

iv. Decompensated cirrhosis patients—It can also be treated while waiting for liver transplantation.

Q.34. What is HBsAg carrier?

Ans. Hepatitis B carrier: HBsAg for >6 months but no evidence of hepatitis clinically, histologically or biochemically.

Q.35. How HBsAg is transmitted vertically?

Ans. During labor admixture of maternal and fetal blood occurs. The virus is transmitted at the time of placental separation. So in case of vaginal delivery, more chance of transmission.

Q.36. How will you manage a case of HBsAg positive pregnancy?

Ans. Managements—

- First see whether it is acute or chronic
- If IgM anti-HBc positive, it is acute
- If there is history of jaundice for more than 6 months, it is Chronic
- If chronic, search for whether active or inactive
- If SGPT normal, it is inactive
- If SGPT twice normal, it is active
- If it is active, then look for replicating or nonreplicating by HBeAg
- In HBsAg positive mother, manage baby with immunoglobulin + vaccination immediately after delivery of baby.

Q.37. Against which viruses' vaccine is available?

Ans. HAV, HBV.

Q.38. How can you prevent HBV infection?

Ans. Active—Hepatitis B vaccine

Passive—Hyperimmune serum globulin, within 24 hours, or at most a week, of exposure to infected blood (e.g. needlestick injury, contamination of cuts or mucous membranes).

Q.39. Can you tell about the route of administration, time schedule and booster dose, duration of protection of vaccine?

Ans. Route: IM (deltoid)

Time:

- For slowest response: 0, 1, 2 and 12 months
- For slow response: 0, 1, 6 months and 5 years

Booster dose after 5 years in case of:

- Immunodeficiency
- Hemodialysis
- Persistent exposure.

Duration of protection: At least for 9 years, may be lifelong.

Q.40. Tell Ab response after vaccination?

Ans. 1–3 months after 3rd dose if:

- Ab<10 IU/L: Nonresponder (full dose should be given).
- Ab 10-100 IU/L: Low responder booster dose should be given.
- Ab> 100 IU/L: High responder.

Q.41. Which group of patient couldn't achieve the protection?

Ans. Group of patient couldn't achieve the protection are:

- Immunocompromised
- Age>50
- Overweight
- HIV+
- Genetics: HLA B8+
- Smoker.

Q.42. What are the other causes of ineffectiveness of vaccine?

Ans. Fault in maintenance of cold chain of the vaccine—Frozen vaccine should be kept in deep freeze 2–8 degrees.

Faulty technique.

Q.43. What is the presentation of hepatitis C virus infection?

Ans. Chronic liver disease.

Q. 44. Does hepatitis C virus cause acute hepatitis?

Ans. Very rare.

Q.45. What is the management of hepatitis C virus infection?

Ans. Managements—

i. The treatment of choice is pegylated α-interferon given weekly subcutaneously, together with oral ribavirin.

ii. Liver transplantation.

Q.46. What do you mean by CLD?

Ans. CLD means chronic liver disease.

Q.47. Which diseases are included in CLD?

Ans. Diseases included in CLD are:
- Chronic hepatitis
- Cirrhosis of liver.

Q.48. Define cirrhosis?

Ans. Diffuse process with fibrosis and nodule formation following hepatocellular necrosis and change in vascular architecture.

Q.49. What are the histological components of cirrhosis?

Ans.
- Inflammatory necrosis of hepatocyte replaced by fibrous tissue
- Regenerative nodule must be present
- Loss of architecture.

NB: These 3 components are essential to have cirrhosis.

Q.50. Classify cirrhosis.

Ans.
1. *Morphological classification*:
   a. Micronodular (<3 mm): This is alcoholic with liver cell failure and minimal portal hypertension regaining.
   b. Macronodular (>3 mm): Following chronic HBV hepatitis with liver failure and portal hypertension progressing.
2. *Etiological classification*:
   - Chronic viral hepatitis (B+/-D or C)
   - Alcohol
   - Drugs: Methotrexate, methyl dopa
   - Nonalcoholic fatty liver disease
   - Immune.
     - Primary sclerozing cholangitis
     - Autoimmune liver disease
   - Biliary
     - Primary biliary cirrhosis
     - Secondary biliary cirrhosis
     - Cystic fibrosis.
   - Genetic
     - Hemochromatosis
     - Wilson's disease
     - α1-antitrypsin deficiency.

   - Cryptogenic (unknown-15%)
   - Chronic venous outflow obstruction
3. *Clinical classification*:
   - Compensated cirrhosis: Cirrhosis without any evidence of decompensation.
   - Decompensated cirrhosis: As evidenced by ascites, increasing jaundice and encephalopathy.

Q.51. What are the common causes of cirrhosis of liver?

Ans. The common causes of cirrhosis of liver are:
- Alcohol
- Virus (Hepatitis B+/-D, Hepatitis C)
- Drugs
- Autoimmune.

Q.52. What are the presentations of cirrhosis of liver?

Ans.
i. Asymptomatic: Diagnosed incidentally at ultrasound or at surgery.
ii. Nonspecific symptoms:
   - Weakness, fatigue
   - Muscle cramps
   - Weight loss
   - Low-grade fever
   - Nonspecific digestive syndrome: Anorexia, nausea, vomiting, upper abdominal discomfort.
iii. Isolated hepatomegaly or splenomegaly.
iv. Features of hepatocellular failure: Jaundice, and encephalopathy.
v. Features due to portal hypertension: Splenomegaly, variceal bleeding (hematemesis, melena).
vi. Features due to complications:
   - Spontaneous bacterial peritonitis
   - Hepatorenal syndrome
   - Hepatopulmonary syndrome
   - HCC.

Q.53. What is the pathogenesis of clinical features of cirrhosis of liver?

Ans.
i. Features of hepatocellular failure: Jaundice, and encephalopathy.
ii. Features due to portal hypertension: Splenomegaly, variceal bleeding (hematemesis, melena).

iii. Combined hepatocellular failure and portal hypertension— Ascites.

Q.54. What are the features of hepatocellular insufficiency?

Ans. Features of hepatocellular insufficiency are:
- Jaundice
- Ascites
- Circulatory changes: Spider telangiectasis
- Palmar erythema
- Cyanosis
- Endocrine changes:
  - Loss of libido and hair loss
  - Men: Gynecomastia, testicular atrophy, and impotence
  - Women: Breast atrophy, and menstrual irregularity

Hemorrhagic tendencies: Bruise, purpura, and epistaxis.

Q.55. What are the features of portal hypertension?

Ans. Features of portal hypertension are:
- Splenomegaly
- Collateral vessels
- Variceal bleeding
- Ascites.

Q.56. What are the complications of CLD?

Ans. Complications of CLD are:
- Ascites
- Spontaneous bacterial peritonitis (SBP)
- Portal hypertension
- Variceal bleeding
- Congestive gastropathy
- Hepatic encephalopathy
- Hepatorenal syndrome
- Hepatopulmonary syndrome
- HCC.

Q.57. What are the cutaneous stigmata of cirrhosis?

Ans. Cutane stigmata of cirrhosis are:
- Leukonychia
- Clubbing
- Palmar erythema
- Dupuytren contracture
- Spider naevi (found above the nipple line, normal 2–3 in 2% population)

- Purpura, ecchymosis
- Generalized pigmentation
- Hepatic facies
- Gynecomastia in male and breast atrophy in female
- Loss of hair.

Q.58. Describe hepatic facies.

Ans. Description of hepatic facies are:
- Muddy complexion
- Shunken eyes
- Prominent zygoma
- Pinched nose
- Thin ala nasi.

Q.59. What are the signs of decompensation of cirrhosis?

Ans. Signs of decompensation of cirrhosis are:
- Increasing jaundice
- Ascites +/– edema
- Encephalopathy
- Fetor hepaticus.

Q.60. What are the investigations done in cirrhosis of liver?

Ans. Investigations are:
- Liver function test
- USG of hepatobiliary system including pancreas: Nonhomogenous coarse parenchymal echotexture is found in liver cirrhosis. Ascites, hepatosplenomegaly may be found.
- Viral markers.
- Ascitic fluid study if ascites present.
- Upper GI endoscopy.
- Liver biopsy (relatively contraindicated in ascites)– Confirmatory.

Q.61. What are the principles of management of cirrhosis?

Ans. Principles of management of cirrhosis are:
- Maintenance of nutrition
- Avoidance of further injury to the liver
- Treatment of causes
- Prevention and treatment of complications
- Liver transplantation in suitable cases.

Q.62. How can you treat a case of CLD?

Ans. Treatment of CLD—
- Nutrition—Protein intake is encouraged, normal requirement is 1 gm/kg/body weight. In acute hepatic

encephalopathy/fulminant hepatic failure, total protein restriction for 5–7 days.
- Avoidance of further injury to the liver.
- Vaccination of other hepatotropic virus A and B.
- Avoidance of hepatotoxic drugs.
- Alcohol avoidance.
- All elective surgeries should be avoided except life-saving surgeries.
- Treatment of causes:
  - Viral hepatitis—Antiviral therapy
  - Alcoholic cirrhosis—Abstinence
  - Wilson's disease—Penicillamine
  - Hemochromatosis—Venesection
  - Primary biliary cirrhosis—Ursodeoxycholic acid
- Prevention and treatment of complications
- Liver transplantation in suitable cases.

Q.63. What is ascites?

Ans. Ascites is the accumulation of free fluid in the peritoneal cavity.

Q.64. What are the causes of ascites?

Ans. Causes of ascites are:
- Cirrhosis of liver
- Cardiac failure
- Intra-abdominal malignancy
- Nephrotic syndrome
- Abdominal tuberculosis
- Others, e.g. malnutrition
- Protein losing enteropathy
- Pancreatitis
- Hypothyroidism.

Q.65. What are the most common causes of ascites?

Ans. The most common causes are:
- Malignant disease
- Cirrhosis
- Heart failure.

Q.66. How much ascites fluid is necessary to detect clinically?

Ans. It depends on the contour of the body. Usually 1L but may be 2 L if obese.

Q.67. How will you differentiate exudative and transudative ascites?

Ans. Ascites is called exudative when ascites protein concentration is above 25 gm/L or a SAAG of less than 11 gm/L and transudative with a total protein concentration below 25 gm/L or a SAAG of more than 11 gm/L.

Q.68. What do you mean by SAAG?

Ans. SAAG: Serum-ascites Albumin Gradient

=Serum albumin conc—Ascites fluid albumin conc.

NB: If the gap is >11 gm/L then it is due to portal hypertension.

A gradient of more than 11 gm/L is 96% predictive that ascites is due to portal hypertension.

Q.69. What is the type of ascites in cirrhosis of liver?

Ans. Transudative ascites.

Q.70. What are the causes of transudative ascites?

Ans. Transudative causes (protein < 25 gm/L) are:

- CCF
- Cirrhosis of liver
- Nephrotic syndrome
- Hypothyroidism
- Hypoproteinemia due to any cause.

Q.71. What are the causes of exudative ascites?

Ans. Exudative causes (protein > 25 gm/L) are:

- Tubercular peritonitis
- Intra-abdominal malignancy
- Pancreatitis.

Q.72. What are the common causes of cirrhotic ascites?

Ans. Common causes of cirrhotic ascites are:

- Avoid salt and water retention
- Portal hypertension
- Hypoalbuminemia
- Secondary aldosteronism
- Slippage of hepatic lymph.

Q.73. What are the principles of treatment of cirrhotic ascites?

Ans. Principles of treatment are:

- Restriction of physical activity

- Salt restriction (cornerstone of management)
- Fluid restriction if serum Na is <125 mmol/L
- Diuretics
- Paracentesis.

Q.74. How can you treat ascites?

Ans. 1. General measures

i. Bed rest—Increase venous return—Increase cardiac output and peripheral circulation—Increase renal circulation and GFR—Increase micturation and fluid excretion.

ii. Salt restriction.

iii. No need of fluid restriction unless serum Na is < 125 mmol/L (i.e. in hyponatremia).

2. Diuretics: Combination of K^+ sparing (spironolactone maximum dose 400 mg, amiloride) and loop diuretics (frusemide maximum dose160) in ratio of 5:2 normally
3. Therapeutic abdominal paracentesis
4. Peritoneovenous shunt (LeVeen shunt)
5. TIPSS.

Q.75. What types of diuretics are used in CLD? Why?

Ans. Spironolactone or combination of spironolactone and frusemide are used in CLD. Because (i) to avoid hypokalemia which may precipitate encephalopathy and (ii) to get the highest efficacy.

Q.76. When diuretics should be stopped?

Ans. Diuretics should be stopped when—

- Ascites is controlled
- Encephalopathy develops
- Serum Na < 120 mmol/L
- Serum creatinine rises.

Q.77. When fluid will be restricted in case of CLD?

Ans. Fluid intake should be restricted when serum Na is < 125 mmol/L (i.e. in hyponatremia).

Q.78. What are the rationalities of treatment of ascites?

Ans. The rationalities of treatment of ascites are:

- To improve the well-being of the patient
- To improve the ascites-related complications mainly SBP
- To prevent development of umbilical hernia.

Q.79. What is refractory ascites and mention its type?

Ans. When highest dose of combination of diuretics (400 mg/day spironolactone and 160 mg/day frusemide), salt restriction fails to control ascites, then it is called refractory ascites.

- Type1—Diuretics resistant refractory ascites
- Type 2—Diuretic intractable refractory ascites.

Q.80. What is the treatment of refractory ascites?

Ans. Treatment of refractory ascites are:

- Therapeutic paracentesis
- LeVeen shunt
- TIPPS
- Ascites ultrafiltration and reinfusion so that effective circulatory volume is not reduced.

Q.81. What are the complications of ascites?

Ans. The complications of ascites are:

- Infection—SBP
- Renal failure
- Abdominal hernia and divarication of recti
- Mesenteric venous thrombosis.

Q.82. What is hepatic encephalopathy?

Ans. It is a neuropsychiatric syndrome caused by liver disease.

Q.83. Which criteria should be present to diagnose hepatic encephalopathy?

Ans. Criteria are—

i. Evidence of acute/chronic liver disease
ii. Evidence of neuropsychiatric manifestation
iii. No evidence of structural abnormality in brain
iv. No other cause of neuropsychiatric abnormality is detected.

Q.84. What are the predisposing factors of hepatic encephalopathy?

Ans. The predisposing factors of hepatic encephalopathy are:

- Uremia: Spontaneous, diuretic induced
- Drugs: Sedatives, hypnotics
- GI bleeding
- Excess dietary protein
- Constipation/diarrhea
- Paracentasis (if >3.5L)

- Hypokalemia
- Infection
- Trauma/surgery
- Portosystemic shunts.

Q.85. Tell the grading of hepatic encephalopathy.

Ans.

Clinical grade	Clinical signs
Grade 1	Poor concentration, slurred speech, slow mentation, and disordered sleep rhythm
Grade 2	Drowsy but easily rousable, occasional aggressive behavior, and lethargic.
Grade 3	Marked confusion, drowsy, sleepy but responds to pain and voice, and gross disorientation.
Grade 4	Unresponsive to voice, may or may not respond to painful stimuli, and unconscious.

Q.86. Which signs will you expect in hepatic encephalopathy?

Ans. Signs are:
- Flapping tremor (asterixis)
- Constructional apraxia
- Hyperreflexia and bilateral extensor plantar responses
- Fetor hepaticus.

Q.87. Is flapping tremor present in every case?

Ans. No, it is found in Grade II and III encephalopathy.

Q.88. What are the principles of management of hepatic encephalopathy?

Ans. The principles of management of hepatic encephalopathy are:
- To treat or remove precipitating causes
- To suppress the production of neurotoxins by bacteria in the bowel.

Q.89. Tell the management of hepatic encephalopathy?

Ans. The management of hepatic encephalopathy are:
- Identify precipitants and correct or treat them
- Dietary protein restriction is rarely needed

- Evacuate and sterilize bowel—Lactulose (15–30 mL 8-hourly).The dose is increased gradually until the bowels are moving twice daily.

  Broad spectrum antibiotics (Rifaximin 550 mg twice daily or Metronidazole (200 mg four times daily) is also effective in the acute situation.

  Neomycin should be avoided.
- Stop or reduce diuretic therapy.
- Maintain nutrition with adequate calories, given if necessary via a fine-bore nasogastric tube, and do not restrict protein for more than 48 hours. Give intravenous fluids as necessary (beware of too much sodium).
- Treat any infection.
- Increase protein in the diet to the limit of tolerance as the encephalopathy improves)
- Liver transplantation.

Q.90. What is the mechanism of action of lactulose in hepatic encephalopathy?

Ans. The mechanism of actions are:
- It produces an osmotic laxative effect
- It reduces the pH of the colonic content
- It, thereby limits colonic ammonia absorption
- It promotes the incorporation of nitrogen into bacteria.

Q.91. What are the differential diagnoses of hepatic encephalopathy?

Ans. Differential diagnosis are:
- Intracranial bleeding (subdural, and extradural hematoma)
- Drug or alcohol intoxication
- Delirium tremens/alcohol withdrawal
- Wernicke encephalopathy
- Primary psychiatric disorders
- Hypoglycemia
- Neurological Wilson's disease
- Postictal state.

Q.92. What are the components of scoring in Child-Pugh classification of prognosis in cirrhosis?

Ans. The components are:
- Encephalopathy

- Bilirubin (μmol/L)
- Albumin (gm/L)
- Prothrombin time (seconds prolonged)
- Ascites.

Q.93. Tell the 5 year and 10 year prognosis as per Child-Pugh classification of prognosis in cirrhosis?

Ans. Add the individual scores: < 7 = Child's A, 7–9 = Child's B, > 9 = Child's C.

Child-Pugh grade	Survival (%) 5 years	10 years
A	45	25
B	20	7
C	20	0

Q.94. Define portal hypertension?

Ans. It is defined as a portal venous pressure above 7 mm Hg (normal; 2–5mm of Hg).

Q.95. When do clinical features or complications develop in portal hypertension?

Ans. Clinical features or complications develop usually when the portal venous pressure exceeds 12 mmHg.

Q.96. What are the mechanisms of developing portal hypertension?

Ans. Mechanisms are:

- Increased portal blood flow
- Increased resistance in the liver (liver architecture is lost – Increase
  Resistance –Less blood flow through liver).

Q.97. What are the common causes of portal hypertension?

Ans. Common causes of portal hypertension are:

- Cirrhosis
- Schistosomiasis
- Portal vein thrombosis
- Budd-Chiari syndrome
- Veno-occlusive disease.

Q.98. What are the clinical features of portal hypertension?

Ans. Clinical features of portal hypertension are:

- Splenomegaly (cardinal feature)

- Variceal bleeding
- Ascites
- Formation of collaterals like caput medusa
- Fetor hepaticus: Results from portosystemic shunting of blood which allows mercaptans to pass directly to lungs.

Q.99. What are the complications of portal hypertension?

Ans. Complications of portal hypertension are:
- Variceal bleeding: Esophageal, gastric, other (rare)
- Congestive gastropathy
- Hypersplenism
- Ascites
- Iron deficiency anemia
- Renal failure
- Hepatic encephalopathy.

Q.100. What is the management of portal hypertension?

Ans. Management of portal hypertension are:
- Treatment is usually directed to specific complications.
- Treatment of underlying cause
- For reduction of portal hypertension
  Tab. Propranolol 80–160 mg/day
  TIPS may be advised.

Q.101. What is the emergency management of variceal bleeding?

Ans. Emergency management of bleeding—

Management	Reason
i. 0.9% saline (1–2 L)	Extracellular volume replacement
ii. Vasopressor (terlipressin)	Reduces portal pressure, acute bleeding and risk of early rebleeding
iii. Prophylactic antibiotics (Cephalosporin IV)	Reduces incidence of SBP
iv. Emergency endoscopy	Confirm variceal rather than ulcer bleed
v. Variceal band ligation	To stop bleeding
vi. Proton pump inhibitor	To prevent peptic ulcers
vii. Phosphate enema and/or lactulose	To prevent hepatic encephalopathy

Q.102. How can you prevent recurrent bleeding?

Ans. Prevention of recurrent bleeding are:
- Drugs: Nonselective β-blocker propranolol
- Endoscopic treatment
  - Scleorotherapy
  - Banding
- TIPSS
- Portosystemic shunt surgery.

Q.103. How can you prevent initial variceal bleeding?

Ans. Prophylaxis for initial variceal bleeding are:
- Propranolol
- Endoscopic band ligation.

Q.104. A patient got admitted in the hospital with jaundice; suddenly he developed unconsciousness, what are the probable causes?

Ans. The probable causes are:
- Acute hepatic failure
- Hepatic encephalopathy on decompensated cirrhosis
- Hypoglycemia in hepatitis patient
- Other causes of coma.

Q.105. What is acute (fulminating) hepatic failure?

Ans. Development of hepatic encephalopathy within 12 weeks of onset of jaundice in patient with no history of liver disease.

Q.106. What is fulminant hepatic failure?

Ans. This is defined as severe hepatic failure in which encephalopathy develops in under 2 weeks in a patient with a previously normal liver.

Q.107. What are the features of FHF?

Ans. Features of FHF are:
- Hepatic encephalopathy
- Cerebral edema
- Fever, vomiting, hypotension and hypoglycemia
- Bleeding from different sites
- Jaundiced patient with a small liver
- Fetor hepaticus is common, but ascites and splenomegaly are rare.
- The mental state varies from slight drowsiness, confusion and disorientation

(Grades I and II) to unresponsive coma (Grade IV) with convulsions.

Q.108. What are the principles of management of FHF?

Ans. i. There is no specific treatment, but patients should be managed in a specialized unit.

ii. Supportive therapy—

- For hepatic encephalopathy—As discussed in hepatic encephalopathy
- For cerebral edema—When signs of raised intracranial pressure are present.
  - 20% mannitol (1 gm/kg bodyweight) should be infused intravenously
  - This dose may need to be repeated. Dexamethasone is of no value.

For hypoglycemia, hypokalemia, hypomagnesemia,

- Hypophosphatemia and hypocalcemia should be anticipated and corrected with 10% dextrose infusion, potassium, calcium, phosphate and magnesium.

For coagulopathy—With intravenous vitamin K, platelets.

- Blood or fresh frozen plasma.
- A proton pump inhibitor (PPI) to prevent gastrointestinal bleeding.

Prophylaxis against infection—Broad spectrum antibiotic.

Renal and respiratory failure should be treated as necessary.

iii. Liver transplantation.

Q.109. What are the causes of acute liver failure?

Ans. Causes of acute liver failure are:

1. Viral infections: Hepatitis A, B, E
2. Drugs: Paracetamol
   - Antitubercular drugs
   - Herbal remedies
   - Halothane
   - Ecstasy
3. Wilson's disease
   - Acute fatty liver of pregnancy
   - Shock and cardiac failure

- Budd-Chairi syndrome
- Leptospirosis

4. Cryptogenic: (non A-E hepatitis).

Q.110. Tell the classification of acute liver failure.

Ans.

Types	Time: Jaundice to encephalopathy
Hyperacute	< 7 days
Acute	8–28 days
Subacute	29 days–12 weeks

Q.111. Name some tumors of the liver.

Ans. Benign—Adenoma and hemangioma

Malignant–

Primary—HCC

Secondary—Metastatic.

Q.112. Which tumor is the most common and why?

Ans. Secondary tumor is the most common and because of dual blood supply—Hepatic artery and portal vein.

Q.113. What are the risk factors/causes for HCC?

Ans. Risk factors causes are:

- Chronic hepatitis B and C infection
- Cirrhosis
- Hemochromatosis
- Nonalcoholic fatty liver disease
- Aflatoxin: *Aspergillus flavus*
- Androgenic steroid.

Q.114. What findings do you expect examining the liver?

Ans. Liver is enlarged, hard in consistency, nodular surface, may be tender and bruit may be present on auscultation.

Q.115. What investigations will you do in HCC?

Ans. Investigations are:

- USG of whole abdomen
- Alpha feto-protein (AFP)- positive in 60% of HCC
- Biopsy
- CT, MRI
- Screening for HBV and HCV.

Q.116. How can you screen HCC in cirrhotic patients?

Ans. We can screen HCC in cirrhotic patients by ultrasound scanning and AFP measurements at 3–6 months intervals.

Q.117. How can you differentiate HCC from secondary tumor?

Ans.

Primary	Secondary
• History of cirrhosis, hepatitis B, C infection	• History of primary carcinoma, e.g. ca stomach, 50% source unknown
• Nodule usually single	• Multiple nodules
• Bruit present	• Rub present
• Umbilication absent	• Umbilication present
• Alpha fetoprotein increased	• Alkaline phosphatase increased
• CEA normal	• CEA increased

Q.118. What is the treatment of HCC?

Ans. Treatment of HCC:

i. Surgical treatment:
   - Hepatic resection
   - Hepatic transplantation

ii. Percutaneous ablation
   - TACE – Transarterial chemoembolism
   - TARE– Transarterial radioembolism
   - TACI– Transarterial chemoinfusion

iii. Systemic chemotherapy

NB: The best option is resection and adjuvant chemotherapy (sorafenib).

Q.119. What are the types of liver abscess?

Ans. Types of liver abscess are:
- Amebic liver abscess
- Pyogenic liver abscess
- Hydatid cyst.

Q.120. What is the organism of amebic liver abscess?

Ans. *Entamoeba histolytica* is the organism of amebic liver abscess.

Q.121. How does it enter into the liver?

Ans. *E.histolytica* enters liver through portal vein.

Q.122. In which lobe of liver, abscess is more common and why?

Ans. Abscess is more common in right lobe because of prominent right portal vein and its left branch is angulated at its origin.

Q.123. What are the common presentations of amebic liver abscess?

Ans. Fever and right hypochondriac pain are the common presentations of amebic liver abscess.

Q.124. What would be your examination findings?

Ans. Raised temperature, soft enlarged tender liver, intercostal space tenderness and edema (punch sign +ve) are the examination findings.

Q.125. What are the causes of enlarged tender liver?

Ans. Causes of enlarged tender liver are:
- Viral hepatitis
- CCF
- Liver abscess
- HCC.

Q.126. What are the investigations done in liver abscess?

Ans. The investigations are:
- USG of liver/CT
- CBC—Neutrophilic leukocytosis with high ESR and CRP.
- Aspiration of pus and C/S (in case of amebic liver abscess no parasite is found as it is present in abscess wall).
- Alkaline phosphatase—Increased in 70% cases.
- CFT, ICT (95% sensitive) in amebic liver abscess.

Q.127. What is the color of pus in amebic liver abscess?

Ans. Anchovy sauce.

Q.128. What do you mean by anchovy sauce?

Ans. Chocolate color like the sauce made by small sea fish.

Q.129. How can you treat amebic liver abscess?

Ans. Metronidazole 800 mg 8 hourly for 5 days or 400 mg 8 hourly for 10 days (alternatives are secnidazole, tinidazole), followed by luminal cysticide: Diloxanide furoate 500 mg 8 hourly for 10 days.

Q.130. How can you assess response?

Ans. Clinically—Fever and pain usually subside within 48–72 hours.

Q.131. What are the indications of therapeutic aspiration of liver abscess?

Ans. Indications are:
- Left lobe abscess
- Size>6 cm
- Impending rupture
- Not responding to medical therapy.

Q.132. What are the causes of hectic rise of temperature (fever with chills and rigor)?

Ans. Causes of hectic rise of temperature are:
- All deep abscess
- UTI/pyelonephritis
- Malaria
- Cholangitis
- Frist episode of pneumococcal pneumonia.

Q.133. Mention organisms causing pyogenic liver abscess.

Ans. The organisms are:
- *E.coli*
- Various streptococci (*Streptococcus milleri*)
- Anaerobes
- Bacteroides.

Q.134. How can you treat pyogenic liver abscess?

Ans. Treatments are:
- Broad spectrum antibiotics—Combination of ampicillin, gentamicin and metronidazole for minimum 2 weeks.
- Alternatives—Ciprofloxacine, ceftriaxone.
- Drainage of abscess.

Q.135. What are the differences between amebic and pyogenic liver abscess?

Ans. The differences between amebic and pyogenic liver abscess are followings:

Trait	Pyogenic	Amebic
History	History of cholangitis and septicemia appendicitis	History of intestinal amebiasis or amebic dysentery (50%)
Organism	*E.coli* Various streptococci (*Streptococcus milleri*) Anaerobes Bacteroides	*Entamoeba histolytica*
Clinical features	High fever with chills and rigors	Mild to moderate fever
Age	Old age/immune compromised	Not so
Onset	Acute	Insidious
Investigation	50% multiple abscess Neutrophilic leukocytosis, Frank pus	Single abscess 90% Anchovy sauce pus
Treatment	Ampicillin gentamicin and metronidazole (AGM) duration of treatment is more	Metronidazole Diloxanide furoate Duration of treatment is less
Prognosis	More fatal	Less fatal

CHAPTER 5

Hematology

Q.1. What is anemia?

Ans. Anemia is defined as the reduced level of hemoglobin in the blood below the normal range appropriate for age and sex.

Q.2. What are the morphological classifications of anemia?

Ans. The morphological classifications are:
- Microcytic hypochromic anemia
- Normocytic normochromic anemia
- Macrocytic anemia.

Q.3. What are the etiological classifications of anemia?

Ans. The etiological classifications are:
- Blood loss anemia
- Hemolytic anemia
- Dyserythropoietic anemia.

Q.4. What are the causes of microcytic hypochromic anemia?

Ans. Causes of microcytic hypochromic anemia are:
- Iron deficiency anemia
- Thalassemia
- Sideroblastic anemia
- Anemia of chronic diseases.

Q.5. A 25-year-old man presents with mild anemia with microcytosis and hypochromia on PBF but not responding to adequate iron therapy. What are you thinking?

Ans. Diagnoses may be:

- Continued blood loss
- Thalassemia minor.

Q.6. What investigation would you suggest?

Ans. Suggested investigation is Hb electrophoresis.

Q.7. What are the causes of dyserythropoietic anemia?

Ans. The causes are:

- Lack of iron, vitamin B_{12} or folate
- Hypoplasia
- Invasion by malignant cells
- Renal failure.

Q.8. What is the most common cause of anemia in female of Bangladesh?

Ans. Iron deficiency is the most common cause of anemia in female of Bangladesh.

Q.9. What is the most common cause of anemia?

Ans. Iron deficiency is the most common cause of anemia.

Q.10. What are the common causes of iron deficiency anemia?

Ans. The common causes are:

- Hookworm infestation.
- Gastrointestinal blood loss—Peptic ulceration, gastritis, occult gastric or colorectal malignancy, inflammatory bowel disease.
- In women of childbearing age, menstrual blood loss, repeated pregnancy and breastfeeding.

Q.11. What are the main causes of iron deficiency anemia worldwide?

Ans. Hookworm and schistosomiasis are the main causes of iron deficiency anemia worldwide.

Q.12. What are the clinical features of anemia?

Ans. **Common symptoms**

- Weakness
- Lassitude
- Tiredness
- Effort intolerance
- Exertional dyspnea
- Chest pain
- Palpitation

- Headache
- Paresthesia.

Common signs

- Pallor
- Peripheral edema
- Cardiac dilatation.

Q.13. What are the specific features of iron deficiency anemia?

Ans. Unusual symptom—Picca, i.e. craving for unusual food, e.g. coal, earth.

Signs—Koilonychia, angular stomatitis and pale smooth tongue.

Q.14. Please tell the findings of PBF in iron deficiency anemia?

Ans. PBF shows—

RBC—Microcytic hypochromic with poikilocytosis, anisocytosis, presence of few target cells

WBC—Normal

Platelet—Normal.

Q.15. What is the confirmatory test for iron deficiency anemia?

Ans. Iron profile is the confirmatory test for iron deficiency anemia.

Q.16. What are the expected findings?

Ans. Findings are:

- Serum ferritin is reduced
- Serum iron is reduced
- TIBC is increased
- Percent saturation reduced.

Q.17. How can you treat iron deficiency anemia due to hookworm?

Ans. Treatment of anemia—

If severe anemia (Hb<6 gm%), blood transfusion. In mild to moderate anemia-iron therapy—Ferrous sulfate 200 mg three times daily for 3–6 months.

Treatment for hookworm—A single dose of albendazole (400 mg).

Q.18. How can you assess response to treatment?

Ans. i. Clinical improvement.
ii. The hemoglobin should rise by 1 g/dL every 7–10 days.
iii. Reticulocyte response will be evident within a week.

Q.19. Why iron therapy is for 3–6 months?

Ans. Iron therapy is for 3–6 months to replenish the iron store.

Q.20. What is the daily requirement of iron?

Ans. Daily requirements: Male: 0.5–1 mg/day.
Menstruating woman:1–3 mg/day.

Q.21. How does hookworm enter into the body?

Ans. Hookworm enters into the body by penetrating skin.

Q.22. How does hookworm cause anemia?

Ans. Hookworm causes iron deficiency anemia by ingesting blood and also causing blood loss from oozing.

Q.23. What are the common side effects of iron therapy?

Ans. GI irritation, constipation, black tongue and stool are the common side effects.

Q.24. Can you tell name of a syndrome associated with iron deficiency?

Ans. Plummer-Vinson syndrome is associated with iron deficiency.

Q.25. What are the components of Plummer-Vinson syndrome?

Ans. The components are:
- Iron deficiency anemia
- Koilonychia
- Dysphagia.

Q.26. What is macrocyte?

Ans. When RBC size is more than 96 fL, it is called macrocytes.

Q.27. Classify macrocytic anemia?

Ans. Classifications of macrocytic anemia are:
- Megaloblastic: Vitamin B_{12} or folate deficiency
- Normoblastic: CLD, hypothyroidism, pregnancy, and alcoholism.

Q.28. Mention the causes of Vit B_{12} deficiency?

Ans. Dietary deficiency in strict vegans

Gastric factors: Gastric surgery and pernicious anemia
Small bowel factors:
- Ileal disease or resection
- Bacterial over growth
- Tropical sprue
- Fish tapeworm.

Q.29. What is pernicious anemia?

Ans. This is an autoimmune disorder in which the gastric mucosa is atrophic, with loss of parietal cells causing intrinsic factor deficiency. In the absence of intrinsic factor, less than 1% of dietary vitamin B_{12} is absorbed leading to megaloblastic anemia.

Q.30. What are the causes of folate deficiency?

Ans. Causes of folate deficiency are:
- Diet—Poor intake of vegetables
- Drugs—Phenytoin, methotrexate, and OCP
- Increased demand—Pregnancy and lactation
- Malabsorption—Celiac disease, Crohn's disease, partial gastrectomy, and cancer
- Alcohol excess.

Q.31. Please tell the sources of vitamin B_{12}.

Ans. Mainly animal protein origin—
- Richest—Kidney, liver, and heart
- Moderate—Meat, fish, egg, cheese, and milk
- Vegetables contain no vitamin B_{12}.

Q.32. Please tell the sources of folic acid.

Ans. Richest—
- Leafy green vegetables
- Liver, kidney, and yeast.

Moderate—Meat, nut, cereals, and milk.

Q.33. Please tell the daily requirement of vitamin B_{12} and folic acid.

Ans. Adult daily requirement: Vitamin B_{12}— 2–4 µg
Folic acid— 200 µg

Q.34. Where is the site of vitamin B_{12} absorption?

Ans. Ileum is the site of vitamin B_{12} absorption.

Q.35. How many years are required to develop vitamin B_{12} deficiency if no vitamin is taken?

Ans. 3 years.

Q.36. Please tell the neurological manifestations of vitamin B_{12} deficiency?

Ans. Neurological manifestations are:
- Peripheral neuropathy
- Subacute combined degeneration of the spinal cord
- Dementia
- Optic atrophy
- Autonomic neuropathy.

Q.37. Which tracts are involved in SCD of spinal cord?

Ans. Tracts involved in SCD of spinal cord are:
- Posterior column—Diminished vibration and proprioception
- Corticospinal tracts— Upper motor neuron.

Q.38. Which deficiency is more common: vitamin B_{12} or folic acid?

Ans. Folic acid deficiency is more common because—
- Folic acid is more destroyed during cooking
- Daily requirement is more
- Vitamin B_{12} is stored in liver for long time than folate.

Q.39. What are the findings in peripheral blood film in megaloblastic anemia?

Ans. Findings are:
- Macrocytosis, poikilocytosis
- Hypersegmented nucleus in neutrophils
- Red cell fragmentation.

Q.40. Please tell the name of the test used to detect vit B_{12} malabsorption.

Ans. Schilling test.

Q.41. How can you manage megaloblastic anemia?

Ans. Management of megaloblastic anemia—

i. Supportive measures—
- Blood transfusion if severe anemia.

ii. Specific measure—Administration of vitamin B_{12} or folic acid
- Vitamin B_{12} deficiency
  - Hydroxycobalamin 1000 μg IM in five doses 2 or 3 days apart.
  - Maintenance therapy —1000 μg every 3 months for life.
- Folate deficiency

- Oral folic acid 5 mg daily for 3 weeks will treat acute deficiency.
- Maintenance therapy— 5 mg once weekly.

NB: The use of folic acid alone in the presence of vitamin B_{12} deficiency may result in worsening of neurological defects.

Q.42. What is aplastic anemia?

Ans. Aplastic anemia is a disorder characterized by simultaneous presence of anemia, leukopenia, and thrombocytopenia due to hypoplasia of bone marrow.

Q.43. What are the causes of aplastic anemia?

Ans. Primary:

- Idiopathic aplastic anemia
- Congenital: Fanconi's anemia.

Secondary:

- Drugs:
  - Cytotoxic drug
  - Antibiotics: Chlormphenicol, sulphonamide
  - Antirheumatics: Penicillamine, gold
  - Antithyroid
  - Anticonvulsants
  - Immunosuppressive drugs: Azathioprine
- Chemicals
  - Benzenes and insecticides like DDT, OPC
- Radiation
- Viral hepatitis
- Pregnancy
- Paroxysmal nocturnal hemoglobinuria.

Q.44. What are the clinical features of aplastic anemia?

Ans. i. Features of anemia
  - Pallor, easy tiredness, exertional dyspnea, chest pain and palpitations

ii. Features of thrombocytopenia
  - Macular or maculopapular spot on skin and/or mucous membrane

iii. Features of leukopenia
  - Fever and sore throat.

No lymphadenopathy, hepatosplenomegaly and bony tenderness.

Q.45. What are the criteria of severe aplastic anemia?

Ans. Criteria are:

- Neutrophil: < 500/mm^3 (in very severe cases it is < 200 mm^3)
- Platelet: < 2000/ mm^3
- Reticulocyte: <1%
- Cellularity: <20%.

Q.46. What are the diagnostic criteria of aplastic anemia?

Ans. Diagnostic criteria are:

- Evidence of anemia, infection and petechiae/purpura at least 2 of these 3 (pancytopenia).
- No generalized lymphadenopathy except local nodes and no hepatosplenomegaly.

Q.47. What are the abdominal findings of aplastic anemia?

Ans. No abnormal findings.

Q.48. Please tell PBF and bone marrow findings of aplastic anemia.

Ans. PBF findings—Pancytopenia

Bone marrow finding—Aplasia or hypoplasia (reduced cellularity).

Q.49. What is the treatment of aplastic anemia?

Ans.

i. Supportive treatment:
   - Correction of anemia by blood transfusion
   - Control of infection with antibiotics
   - Correction of thrombocytopenia by platelet/fresh blood transfusion
   - In case of menorrhagia uninterrupted OCP.

ii. Marrow stimulating agents like oxymetholone, anabolic steroid, methyl prednisolone (to get desired action of these drugs 6 months is required).

iii. Bone marrow transplantation for patients under 30 years of age (curative treatment). In older patients, immunosuppressive therapy with cyclosporine and antithymocyte globulin.

iv. Treatment of complications—

   Advice

- Avoid IM injections–As chance of formation of muscle hematoma.
- Elective surgeries should be postponed.
- Barrier nursing.

Q.50. What is the treatment for fever with aplastic anemia?

Ans. Immediate institution of broad-spectrum parenteral antibiotics (e.g. meropenem, piperacillin or tozabactam).

Q.51. What is pancytopenia? What are its causes?

Ans. Pancytopenia means the presence of anemia, leukopenia and thrombocytopenia. Causes are—

i. Bone marrow failure.

ii. Hypoplastic/aplastic anemia: Inherited, idiopathic, viral, drugs.

iii. Bone marrow infiltration
- Acute leukemia
- Myeloma
- Lymphoma
- Carcinoma
- Myelodysplastic syndromes.

iv. Ineffective hematopoiesis
- Megaloblastic anemia

v. Peripheral pooling/destruction
- Hypersplenism
- Systemic lupus erythematosus (SLE).

Q.52. A 12-year-old boy presents with tiredness with history of multiple blood transfusion. On examination patient is anemic, have jaundice and splenomegaly. What is your diagnosis?

Ans. Hereditary hemolytic anemia.

Q.53. What are the triad of hemolytic anemia?

Ans. Triad of hemolytic anemia are anemia, jaundice, and splenomegaly.

Q.54. Define hereditary hemolytic anemia.

Ans. It is a group of inherited disorders characterized by excessive RBC destruction greater than erythropoiesis.

Q.55. What is the normal lifespan of RBC?

Ans. Normal lifespan of RBC is about 120 days.

Q.56. Tell the name of normal hemoglobins with globin chains.

Ans.

Normal hemoglobins	Types	Structure
Adult	Hb A	$\alpha_2\,\beta_2$
	Hb A_2	$\alpha_2\delta_2$
Fetal	Hb F	$\alpha_2\gamma_2$

Q.57. Please tell the percentage of different hemoglobins at birth.

Ans. Hb A 97%
Hb A_2< 2%
Fetal Hb<1%.

Q.58. Please tell the name of some hereditary hemolytic anemia.

Ans. The name of some hereditary hemolytic anemia are thalassemia, sickle cell anemia, hereditary spherocytosis, HbE disease, and thalassemia-E disease.

Q.59. What are more common in this subcontinent?

Ans. HbE disease, thalassemia-E disease and thalassemia are more common in this subcontinent.

Q.60. What is thalassemia?

Ans. It is an inherited impairment of Hb production in which there is partial or complete failure to synthesis a specific type of globin chain.

Q.61. What is the mode of inheritance of thalassemia?

Ans. Autosomal recessive disorder is the mode of inheritance of thalassemia.

Q.62. Please tell the clinical features of thalassemia.

Ans. Clinical features are:

- Failure to thrive (slow growth)
- Recurrent bacterial infection
- Thalassemic facies (hemolytic):
  - Frontal and parietal boosing
  - Malar prominence

- Depressed nasal bridge
- Malocclusion of teeth

- Anemia
- Mild jaundice
- Splenomegaly
- Hepatomegaly.

Q.63. What is the diagnostic criteria for hereditary hemolytic anemia?

Ans. Two history-positive family history and repeated blood transfusion history plus three cardinal features—Anemia, jaundice and splenomegaly.

Q.64. How can you diagnose thalassemia by investigation?

Ans. PBF—Microcytic hypochromic cells, target cells, fragmented RBC (classic).

Hb-electrophoresis

- Minor—HbA_2 increased
- Major—HbF increased

Hb%-reduced.

X-ray skull—Widening of diploic space, thinning of cuticle, thickening of trabeculae, hair on end appearance, Iron profile: Serum iron, ferritin, TIBC and percentage saturation are all normal.

If repeated blood transfusions then: Serum iron, ferritin, % saturation are all increased and TIBC is decreased.

Others (to see complications): CXR, ECG, Echo, blood sugar, USG of whole abdomen.

Q.65. Which is confirmatory investigation?

Ans. Hb-electrophoresis is confirmatory investigation.

Q.66. Please tell the treatment of thalassemia?

Ans. Treatment of thalassemia—

i. Hemopoietic support (if necessary): Blood transfusion is done to keep Hb above 10 gm/dL.
ii. Folic acid 5 mg daily for lifelong (relative deficiency occurs due to increase demand for erythropoiesis and maturation of RBC).
iii. Iron therapy forbidden iron chelating agent: Desferrioxamine (if indicated).

iv. Allogenic bone marrow transplantation is curative. (done in case of thalassemia major).
v. Splenectomy.
vi. Evaluation of patient to see any complication if present, treatment should be given.
vii. Gene therapy (latest).
viii. Counseling.

Q.67. What are the indications of splenectomy in thalassemia?

Ans. Indications of splenectomy in thalassemia are:

- Features of hypersplenism
- Significant mechanical pressure
- Increased frequency of blood transfusion
- Splenic rupture.

Q.68. What are infectious agents for which splenectomized patients are susceptible?

Ans. Infectious agents are:

- *H.influenzae*
- *S.pneumoniae*
- *N.meningitides*
- Malaria.

Q.69. What are the components of counseling in thalassemia?

Ans. Components are:

- Genetic counseling
- Blood examination before marriage
- Prenatal diagnosis: by chorionic villi sampling or by amniotic fluid study.

Q.70. How frequently is blood transfusion needed?

Ans. 3–4 months interval as RBC lifespan is 120 days.

Q.71. What is iron overload?

Ans. When total body iron is increased is called iron overload.

Q.72. Iron overload anemia occurs in which condition?

Ans. Hereditary hemolytic anemia with repeated blood transfusion.

Q.73. Folic acid supplementation should be given in thalassemia, why?

Ans. There is increased and ineffective erythropoiesis in response causing increased demand of folic acid. So folic acid supplementation is given for lifelong.

Q.74. What are the indications of blood transfusion in thalassemia?

Ans. **Absolute**:

- If Hb less than or equal to 6 mg/dL irrespective of clinical features.
- Hb 6–8 mg/dL with clinical features like chest pain dyspnea and palpitation.

Relative:

- Hb 6.1–8 mg/dL without signs and symptoms
- Hb 8.1–10 with signs and symptoms.

Q.75. What is hypertransfusion and supertransfusion?

Ans. i. Hypertransfusion means blood transfusion to achieve Hb concentration from 11–12 gm/dL.

Its aim is to prevent bony deformity

ii. Supertransfusion means blood transfusion to achieve concentration from 14–15 gm/dL.

Its aim is for intellectual development and growth in first 2 years of life.

Q.76. Please mention the complications of transfusion in thalassemia?

Ans. Immediate:

i. Transfusion reaction:
   - Mismatched blood transfusion
   - Febrile reaction
   - Allergic reaction.

ii. Transmission of disease:
   - Bacterial: Syphilis
   - Viral: Hepatitis B, C and HIV

iii. Thrombophlebitis

iv. Air embolism

v. Volume overload—Causing heart failure

vi. Coagulopathy

vii. Hypercalcemia

viii. Hyperkalemia

ix. Hypokalemia
x. Citrate toxicity
xi. DIC.

Late:
i. Hemosiderosis
ii. Hemochromatosis.

Q.77. Define hemosiderosis and hemochromatosis?

Ans. Hemosiderosis is the iron deposition in intracellular spaces without damaging organs.

Hemochromatosis (iron loading anemia): Hemochromatosis is a disorder of iron storage that results in increased intestinal iron absorption with iron deposition and damage to many tissues.

Q.78. What are the target organs of hemochromatosis?

Ans. Target organs are:
- Heart—Restricted type of cardiomyopathy
- Pancreas—Bronze diabetes
- Liver—Commonly cirrhosis of liver, later HCC
- Joint—Arthropathy, commonly involving 2nd and 3rd metacarpophalangeal joints
- Skin—Leaden gray skin pigmentation due to excessive melanin or bronze callus
- Genitalia—Testicular atrophy, loss of libido, infertility.

Q.79. What are the features of hypersplenism?

Ans. Features are:
- Splenomegaly
- Pancytopenia
- Increase cellularity of bone marrow
- Improvement of blood picture after splenectomy.

Q.80. What is the prerequisite for splenectomy?

Ans.
- Proper indication
- Consent
- Pneumococcal, *Hemophilus influenzae* type B, meningococcal group C and influenza vaccines at least 2–3 weeks before elective splenectomy.

Q.81. What are the causes of death in thalassemia?

Ans. i. Heart failure—
1. *Ischemic cardiomyopathy*: Hypoxia and ischemia cause IHD leading to ischemic cardiomyopathy.

2. *Restrictive cardiomyopathy*: Iron overload leading to hemosiderosis and finally hemochromatosis and develops restrictive cardiomyopathy.

ii. Intercurrent infection.

Q.82. An 8-year-old girl has purpuric spots on different parts of the body and no other abnormal findings. Her platelet count is 70,000/cmm. What is your diagnosis?

Ans. Diagnosis will be idiopathic thrombocytopenic purpura (ITP).

Q.83. What is ITP?

Ans. ITP is an acquired disorder leading to immune-mediated destruction of platelets and possibly inhibition of platelet release from the megakaryocyte.

Q.84. What are the types of ITP?

Ans. Types are—

Acute ITP: It occurs in children, commonly follows an infection, self-limiting.

Chronic ITP: It occurs in adults, insidious onset, chronic course, more commonly affects females, unusual to have history of preceding viral infection.

Q.85. What is the mechanism of ITP?

Ans. ITP is due to autoimmune mechanism mediated by autoantibodies, most often directed against the platelet membrane glycoprotein IIb/IIIa, which sensitize the platelet, resulting in premature removal from the circulation by cells of the reticuloendothelial system.

Q.86. What are the presentations of ITP? Is it common in male or female?

Ans. Purpura, petechiae, and bruises are the presentations of ITP. It is common in female.

Q.87. What is purpura? What are the causes of purpura?

Ans. Purpura is extravasation of blood in skin and mucous membrane which does not blanch on pressure and undergoes progressive color change.

Causes are:

- Idiopathic thrombocytopenic purpura
- DIC
- Viral infection—Dengue fever and EBV

  - Meningococcal septicemia
- Drugs—Aspirin, NSAIDs
  Aplastic anemia
  Acute leukemia.

Q.88. What history would you take?

Ans. – History of bleeding, e.g. purpura and gum bleeding
– History of respiratory infection 2–3 weeks before.

Q.89. How can you differentiate acute ITP from chronic ITP?

Ans.

Acute	Chronic
Occurs in children	Occurs in adults
Occurs in both sex	More common in females
Acute onset	Insidious onset
Self-limiting	Chronic course
Commonly follows respiratory infection	No history of respiratory infection

Q.90. If a patient presents with rash and your suspicion is ITP, which single investigation would you advice?

Ans. Blood for TC, DC, Hb%, ESR, PBF, and platelet count.

Q.91. What is your expectation in ITP?

Ans. Reduced platelet count is the expectation in ITP.

Q.92. What investigation will you do to confirm your diagnosis?

Ans. Bone marrow study.

Q.93. What is your expectation?

Ans. Increased megakaryocytes in bone marrow.

Q.94. If megakaryocytes are decreased, what will you think?

Ans. Bone marrow hypoplasia, infiltration (e.g. leukemia).

Q.95. What is the treatment of ITP?

Ans. i. Supportive:
- Blood transfusion
- Platelet transfusion

ii. Specific:

- Steroids—Oral prednisolone at least 2 weeks followed by tapering over 3–4 weeks
- Dose—Children—2 mg/kg, adult—1mg/kg
- Indications—Moderate to severe purpura, bruising or epistaxis, platelet count less than 10×10^9/L

If fails, then

IV immunoglobulin.

If fails, then

IV immunoglobulin plus steroid

If no response then

Splenectomy

If fails, then

Immunosuppressive therapy—Vincristine, azathioprine, cyclophosphamide, rituximab used in refractory cases, failed to respond to steroid and splenectomy.

Q.96. What are the indications of platelet transfusion in ITP?

Ans. Indications are:

i. Severe bleeding not controlled with steroid—Persistent epistaxis, gastrointestinal bleeding, retinal hemorrhages, intracranial bleeding.

ii. Before splenectomy.

Q.97. What are the indications of splenectomy in ITP?

Ans. i. Chronic cases with two relapses

ii. Life-threatening bleeding not controlled by other means

iii. First 4–5 months of pregnancy when steroid failed to induce remission.

Q.98. What are the indications of OCP in unmarried girl/ medical indications of OCP?

Ans. Indications are:

i. Menorrhagia due to ITP or bleeding disorder or thrombocytopenia due to any cause.

ii. Dysmenorrhea

iii. DUB

iv. Polycystic ovarian syndrome.

Q.99. A 9-year-old boy presents with swelling of right knee joint after a minor trauma. On examination, fluctuation

test is positive but no sign of inflammation. On query patient's father admitted excessive bleeding during circumcision in past. What is your diagnosis?

Ans. Diagnosis is hemophilia.

Q.100. What is the cause of hemophilia?

Ans. Cause of hemophilia is deficiency of factor VIII (classical hemophilia A) or factor IX (Christmas disease hemophilia B).

Q.101. What is the mode of inheritance?

Ans. It is an X-linked recessive disorder.

Q.102. Which history would you take?

Ans. Bleeding history—During circumcision, tooth extraction, and cut injury.

Family history—Maternal aunt and cousin.

Q.103. What investigations are done in hemophilia?

Ans. **Screening test**

- Clotting time—Prolonged
- Bleeding time—Normal
- APTT prolonged
- Prothrombin time—Normal
- Platelet—Normal

Confirmatory test

- Factor VIII assay
- Factor IX assay.

Q.104. Please tell the treatment of hemophilia?

Ans. Treatments are:

- In hemophilia A— IV infusion of factor VIII, if not available fresh blood.
- In hemophilia B— IV infusion of factor IX.
- Rest of the bleeding site by either bed rest or a splint reduces continuing hemorrhage.
- Once bleeding has settled, patient should be mobilized and physiotherapy used to restore strength to the surrounding muscles.

Q.105. Define leukemia.

Ans. Leukemias are malignant disorders of the hematopoietic stem cell compartment, characteristically associated with increased numbers of white cells in the bone marrow and/or peripheral blood.

Q.106. Classify leukemias.

Ans. Leukemias are traditionally classified into four main groups:

- Acute lymphoblastic leukemia (ALL)
- Acute myeloid leukemia (AML)
- Chronic lymphocytic leukemia (CLL)
- Chronic myeloid leukemia (CML).

Q.107. Please tell the clinical features of acute leukemia.

Ans. Clinical features of acute leukemia are:

- Usually abrupt onset.
- Signs of bone marrow failure: Anemia, infection, bleeding constitutional symptoms: Fever, malaise, weakness, tiredness, sweating, anorexia, weight loss.
- Hepatosplenomegaly.
- Lymphadenopathy.
- Bony tenderness.

Q.108. Please tell the blood picture of acute leukemia.

Ans. CBC

- Hb% decrease
- Total count of WBC: 50,000–1 lac
- Differential count: Increase immature cells, blast cells>10%
- ESR increased
- Platelet count decreased.

PBF

- RBC: Normocytic, normochromic, anisocytosis, and poikilocytosis.
- WBC blast cell increased.
- Auer rods in the cytoplasm of blast cells indicates a myeloblastic type of leukemia.
- Platelet: Thrombocytopenia.

Q.109. Please tell the bone marrow findings in acute leukemia.

Ans. Bone marrow findings are:

- Hypercellular bone marrow
- M/E ratio: Increased
- Granulopoiesis: Increased, blast cell>20%

- Erythropoiesis Depressed
- Megakaryopoiesis reduced.

Q.110. What are the principles of treatment of acute leukemia?

Ans. i. Supportive therapy

- Anemia—Anemia is treated with red cell concentrate transfusions. (Hb<10 gm/dL)
- Bleeding—Thrombocytopenic bleeding requires platelet transfusions (Pl<10 × 10^9/L)
- Infection—Aggressive management of infection.
- Fluid and electrolyte imbalance and nutritional maintenance.

ii. Specific therapy.

Q.111. What are the phases of specific therapy?

Ans. There are three phases—

- Remission induction
- Remission consolidation
- Remission maintenance.

Q.112. What are the myeloproliferative disorders?

Ans. Myeloproliferative disorders are:

- CML
- Polycythemia rubra Vera
- Essential thrombocythemia
- Myelofibrosis or myelosclerosis.

Q.113. What are the phases of CML?

Ans. The disease has three phases:

- Chronic phase
- Accelerated phase
- Blast crisis.

Q.114. Which chromosome is responsible for CML?

Ans. Philadelphia (Ph) chromosome is responsible for CML.

Q.115. What is Philadelphia (Ph) chromosome?

Ans. This is a shortened chromosome 22 resulting from a reciprocal translocation of material with chromosome 9.

Q.116. How many patients with CML is Ph chromosome positive?

Ans. 95% patients with CML is Ph chromosome positive.

Q.117. What is the age incidence of CML?

Ans. Between the ages of 30 and 80 years, with a peak incidence at 55 years.

Q.118. What are the common presentations of CML?

Ans. The common presentations are:

- Asymptomatic
- Splenomegaly
- Nonspecific—Anemia, infection, and fatigue.

Q.119. What is the blood picture of CML?

Ans. RBC: Normocytic normochromic anisocytosis poikilocytosis

WBC: The leukocyte count can vary from 10 to 600 × 10^9/L.

Platelet: Increased/normal.

In PBF, the full range of granulocyte precursors from myeloblasts to mature neutrophils is seen but the predominant cells are neutrophils and myelocytes.

Q.120. What is the first line therapy for CML in chronic phase?

Ans. Imatinib is the first line therapy for CML in chronic phase.

Q.121. How does it act?

Ans. Imatinib specifically inhibits BCR ABL tyrosine kinase activity and reduces the uncontrolled proliferation of white cells.

Q.122. Which variety of leukemia is most common?

Ans. Chronic lymphocytic leukemia (CLL) is the most common variety of leukemia.

Q.123. Which is the median age of presentation?

Ans. The median age at presentation is 65–70 years.

Q.124. What are the presentations of CLL?

Ans. The presentations are:

- Asymptomatic—70% diagnosis is made incidentally on a routine FBC.
- Generalized lymphadenopathy
- Anemia, infections,
- Systemic symptoms such as night sweats or weight loss.

Q.125. Which drug is used to treat CLL?

Ans. Chlorambucil is used to treat CLL.

Q.126. A 35-year-male presented to you with generalized lymphadenopathy for 6 months. You found hepatosplenomegaly on examination. What are your differential diagnoses?

Ans. Differential diagnosis are:
- Lymphoma
- Leukemia
- Disseminated tuberculosis.

Q.127. What is generalized lymphadenopathy? Mention the causes of lymphadenopathy?

Ans. When two or more noncontiguous lymph node groups are involved, then it is called generalized lymphadenopathy.

Causes are—

Generalized—
- Viral: Epstein-Barr virus (glandular fever or Burkitt's lymphoma), cytomegalovirus, HIV
- Bacterial: Brucellosis, syphilis
- Protozoal: Toxoplasmosis
- Malignancy: Lymphoma, acute or chronic lymphocytic leukemia
- Inflammatory: Rheumatoid arthritis, SLE, and sarcoidosis.

Localized—
- Infective: Infection in the draining area, acute or chronic, bacterial or viral.
- Malignancy: Secondary metastases, lymphoma (Hodgkin's or non-Hodgkin's lymphoma).

Q.128. What are the types of lymphoma?

Ans. Types are:
- Hodgkin's lymphoma
- Non-Hodgkin's lymphoma.

Q.129. Please tell WHO classification of Hodgkin' lymphoma (HL).

Ans.
i. Nodular lymphocyte-predominant HL
ii. Classical HL
   a. Nodular sclerosing
   b. Mixed cellularity
   c. Lymphocyte—Rich
   d. Lymphocyte—Depleted.

Q.130. Classify non-Hodgkin's lymphoma.

Ans. Classifications are:
- High-grade tumors
- Low-grade tumors.

Q.131. Differentiate non-Hodgkin's lymphoma from Hodgkin's lymphoma?

Ans.

Features	Hodgkin's lymphoma	Non-Hodgkin's lymphoma
Lymph node involvement	Usually localized to single axial group	Peripheral lymph node involvement
Mesenteric lymph node and Waldeyer's ring	Rarely involved	Commonly involved
Lymph node spread	Orderly spread by contiguity	Noncontiguous spread
Extranodal involvement	Less common	More common
Systemic features	Common	Less common
Pel-Ebstein fever	May occur	Does not occur
Pruritis	Common	Less common
Histology	Reed-Sternberg cell	Absent
Prognosis	High cure rate	Low cure rate

Q.132. What is the hallmark of Hodgkin's lymphoma?

Ans. Reed-Sternberg cell is the hallmark of Hodgkin's lymphoma.

Q.133. What is the clinical staging of lymphoma?

Ans.
I. Involvement of a single lymph node region (I) or extralymphatic site (IE).
II. Involvement of two or more lymph node regions (II) or an extralymphatic site and lymph node regions on the same side of (above or below) the diaphragm (IIE).
III. Involvement of lymph node regions on both sides of the diaphragm with (IIIE) or without (III) localized extralymphatic involvement or involvement of the spleen (IIIS) or both (IIISE).

IV. Diffuse involvement of one or more extralymphatic tissues, e.g. liver or bone marrow.

Q.134. What are the modalities of treatment of Hodgkin's lymphoma?

Ans. Modalities are:
- Radiotherapy
- Chemotherapy
- Combined therapy.

Q.135. What is the treatment of Hodgkin's lymphoma?

Ans. i. Radiotherapy
- Stage I and IIA disease.
- After chemotherapy to sites where there was originally bulk disease.
- To lesions causing serious pressure problems.

ii. Chemotherapy
- ABVD (doxorubicin, vinblastine, bleomycin and dacarbazine) therapy every 3–4 weeks for a total of 6–8 cycles. Treatment response is assessed clinically and by repeat CT
  Indications:
  - Stage III and IV
  - All symptomatic patients(All stage B)
  - Stage IIa (>3 lymph node involvement)

iii. Combined therapy.

Q.136. What are the causes of low back pain with increased ESR?

Ans. Causes are:
- Multiple myeloma
- Bony metastasis.

Q.137. Define multiple myeloma?

Ans. It is a neoplastic proliferation of plasma cell that infiltrates the bone marrow and other tissue and produce abnormal Ig that accumulate in blood. It is a plasma cell disorder.

Q.138. What is the most common presentation of multiple myeloma?

Ans. Back pain in elderly patient is the most common presentation of multiple myeloma.

Q.139. How to diagnose multiple myeloma?

Ans. Diagnosis of multiple myeloma requires two of the following three—

i. Increased malignant plasma cells in the bone marrow
ii. Serum and/or urinary paraprotein
iii. Skeletal lytic lesions.

Q.140. How can you treat multiple myeloma?

Ans. i. If patients are asymptomatic, no treatment is required.

ii. Supportive—
- High fluid intake to treat renal impairment and hypercalcemia
- Analgesia for bone pain.
- Bisphosphonates for hypercalcemia and to delay other skeletal related events
- Allopurinol to prevent urate nephropathy.
- Plasmapheresis, as necessary, for hyperviscosity.

iii. Specific therapy—
- Chemotherapy ± bone marrow transplantation
  - In older patients, thalidomide + melphalan + prednisolone.
  - In younger, fitter patients, thalidomide + melphalan + prednisolone + autologous stem-cell transplantation.

Q.141. What are poor prognostic factors?

Ans. Poor prognostic factors are:
- High β_2-microglobulin
- Low albumin
- Low hemoglobin
- High calcium at presentation.

Q.142. What are the blood products used therapeutically?

Ans. Blood products are:

i. Whole blood
ii. Red cell concentrate
iii. Platelet concentrate
iv. Fresh frozen plasma— It is used to replace coagulation factors
v. Cryoprecipitate— It is used to replace fibrinogen
vi. Coagulation factor concentrate— It is to replace factor VIII and factor IX.
vii. IV immunoglobulin— It is used in GBS and ITP.

CHAPTER 6

Renal System

Q.1. What is oliguria?

Ans. When urinary output is less than 300 mL in a day on a normal diet.

Q.2. What is anuria?

Ans. It is the complete absence of urine production for the last 24 hours or less than 30 mL/day.

Q.3. What is polyuria?

Ans. Polyuria means excessive urinary output, i.e. urine volume >3 L/day.

Q.4. What are the causes of polyuria?

Ans. Causes are:

- Excess fluid intake
- Osmotic, e.g. hyperglycemia (DM) and hypercalcemia
- Cranial diabetes insipidus—Idiopathic (50%), mass lesion, trauma, and infection.
- Nephrogenic diabetes insipidus
  - Drugs/toxins, e.g. lithium and diuretics
  - Interstitial renal disease
  - Hypokalemia, hypercalcemia.

Q.5. What is UTI?

Ans. Urinary tract infection (UTI) is defined as multiplication of organisms in the urinary tract. It is usually associated with the presence of neutrophils and $>10^5$ organisms/mL in midstream clean catch morning sample of urine. Exception in pregnancy $>10^4$ organisms/mL as UTI has deleterious effects.

Q.6. How can you collect midstream clean catch morning sample of urine?

Ans. A sterile test tube/container should be taken and patient should be instructed to collect urine during first voiding after overnight sleep and first part of urine flow is allowed to pass and collect the middle part of the stream.

Q.7. What is strangury and dysuria?

Ans. Strangury—Painful urge for micturition but unable to pass urine.
Dysuria—Painful micturition.

Q.8. Tell the criteria for diagnosis of UTI.

Ans. Criteria for diagnosis of bacteriuria are:
Symptomatic young women
$\geq 10^2$ coliform organisms/mL urine plus pyuria (> 10 WCC/mm^3)
Or
$\geq 10^5$ any pathogenic organism/mL urine
Or
any growth of pathogenic organisms in urine by suprapubic aspiration
Symptomatic men
$\geq 10^3$ pathogenic organisms/mL urine
Asymptomatic patients
$\geq 10^5$ pathogenic organisms/mL urine on two occasion.

Q.9. What are the spectrum of presentations of urinary tract infection?

Ans. The spectrum of presentations are:
- Asymptomatic bacteriuria
- Symptomatic acute urethritis and cystitis
- Acute pyelonephritis
- Acute prostatitis
- Septicemia (usually gram-negative bacteria).

Q.10. What do you mean by lower urinary tract infection?

Ans. Lower urinary tract infection includes urethritis and cystitis (urethral and bladder inflammation respectively).

Q.11. What is pyelonephritis?

Ans. The infection to the pelvis and kidney is known as pyelitis or pyelonephritis.

Q.12. What are the common presentations of lower UTI?

Ans. Common presentations are:
- Frequency of micturition by day and night
- Painful voiding (dysuria)
- Suprapubic pain and tenderness
- Hematuria
- Foul smell urine.

Q.13. What are the common features of pyelonephritis?

Ans. Common features of pyelonephritis are:
- Loin pain and tenderness
- Prominent systemic symptoms—Fever with rigors, vomiting and hypotension.

Q.14. What are the organisms responsible for UTI?

Ans. Typical organisms causing UTI in the community—
- *E. coli* (about 75% of infections)
- Proteus spp
- Pseudomonas spp
- Streptococci
- *Staphylococcus epidermidis.*

In hospital—
- *E. coli*
- Klebsiella
- Streptococci.

Q.15. Why is UTI more common in woman?

Ans. Because of—
- The urethra is shorter
- Closer to perineum
- Absence of bactericidal prostatic secretions
- Sexual intercourse may cause minor urethral trauma and transfer bacteria from the perineum into the bladder.

Q.16. What do you mean by complicated and uncomplicated UTI?

Ans. *Uncomplicated UTI* means UTI occurring without any anatomical, physiological and immunological defect. Here, persistent or recurrent infection seldom results in serious kidney damage.

Complicated UTI means UTI occurring with anatomical (e.g.urethral stricture), physiological (e.g.vesicoureteric reflux) or immunological defect (e.g.diabetes). Here, persistent or recurrent infection results in serious kidney damage.

Q.17. What are the types of recurrent infection?

Ans. Relapse and reinfection are the types of recurrent infection.

Q.18. What are relapse and reinfection?

Ans. *Relapse* is diagnosed by recurrence of bacteriuria with the same organism within 7 days of completion of antibacterial treatment and implies failure to eradicate infection.

Reinfection is when bacteriuria is absent after treatment for at least 14 days, usually longer, followed by recurrence of infection with the same or different organisms.

Q.19. What is the treatment for uncomplicated UTI?

Ans. Treatment is started while awaiting urine c/s report

Antibiotic: Amoxicillin 250 mg 8-hourly
Nitrofurantoin 50 mg 6-hourly
Cephalexin 250 mg 6-hourly
Ciprofloxacin 100 mg 12-hourly
Co-amoxiclav 250/125 mg 8-hourly
Duration—3 days in women, 10 days in men.

Q.20. Which prophylactic measures should be taken by women with recurrent urinary infections?

Ans. Prophylactic measures are:

- Fluid intake of at least 2 L/day
- Regular complete emptying of bladder
- Good personal hygiene
- Emptying of the bladder before and after sexual intercourse
- Cranberry juice may be effective.

Q.21. Which drugs would you use to treat UTI in a pregnant lady?

Ans. Drugs are:

- Cefuroxim
- Amoxicillin.

Q.22. What is asymptomatic bacteriuria?

Ans. It is defined as $>10^5$/mL organisms in urine of apparently healthy asymptomatic patients.

Q.23. When treatment is needed in asymptomatic bacteriuria?

Ans. Treatment is usually needed in infants, pregnant women and those with urinary tract abnormalities.

Q.24. What are the causes of hematuria?

Ans. The causes of hematuria are:
- Glomerulonephritis
- Tumor
- Infection
- Infarction
- Cysts in kidney
- Stones.

Q.25. What are the medical causes of hematuria?

Ans. Causes of hematuria are:
- Glomerulonephritis
- Urinary tract infection
- Infective endocarditis
- Infarction
- Benign familial hematuria
- Blood dyscrasia.

Q.26. What are the causes of painless hematuria?

Ans. Causes of painless hematuria are:
- Glomerulonephritis
- Renal tuberculosis
- Infective endocarditis
- Benign familial hematuria
- Blood dyscrasia.

Q.27. What is orthostatic proteinuria?

Ans. Proteinuria occurring after long-standing is called orthostatic proteinuria.

Q.28. How will you perform a heat coagulation test?

Ans. Two-thirds of a test tube is filled with urine. A blue litmus paper is emmersed to test the reaction of urine. If alkaline, a few drops of 5% acetic acid is added to make urine acidic. Then upper portion of urine is heated to boiling and checked.

Q.29. What is normal reaction of urine?

Ans. Normal reaction of urine is acidic.

Q.30. What is interpretation of heat coagulation test?

Ans. After heating if there is cloudiness, it indicates presence of protein or phosphate. A few drops of acetic acid is added and heated again, phosphate will dissolve but protein intensifies.

Q.31. What are the causes of red urine?

Ans. Causes of red urine are:
- Hematuria
- Hemoglobinuria
- Myoglobinuria
- Food dyes
  - For example, anthocyanins (beetroot)
- Drugs

  For example, phenolphthalein—Pink when alkaline

  Senna/other anthraquinones—Orange
  Rifampicin—Orange
  Levodopa—Darkens on standing
  Porphyria—Darkens on standing
  Alkaptonuria
  Bilirubinuria

  For example, obstructive jaundice—Dark.

Q.32. What are the characteristics of glomerular hematuria?

Ans. Characteristics are:
- Dysmorphic RBC
- RBC cast.

Q.33. What are the features of nephritic syndrome?

Ans. Features of nephritic syndrome are:
- Hematuria (red or brown urine)
- Edema and generalized fluid retention
- Hypertension
- Oliguria.

Q.34. What are the features of nephrotic syndrome?

Ans. Features of nephrotic syndrome are:
- Massive proteinuria: Usually > 3.5 gm/24 hours (urine may be frothy)
- Hypoalbuminemia (< 30 gm/L)
- Edema and generalized fluid retention
- Hyperlipidemia.

Q.35. Which glomerulopathies present as nephritic syndrome?

Ans. Glomerulopathies present as nephritic syndrome are:
- Poststreptococcal glomerulonephritis
- Goodpasture's disease (anti-GBM disease)
- IgA nephropathy
- Henoch-Schönlein purpura.

Q.36. Which glomerulopathies present as nephrotic syndrome?

Ans. Glomerulopathies present as nephrotic syndrome are:
- Minimal change nephropathy
- Focal segmental glomerulosclerosis (FSGS)
- Membranous nephropathy
- Diabetic nephropathy
- SLE.

Q.37. Which glomerulopathies present as nephritonephrotic syndrome?

Ans. Glomerulopathies present as nephitonephrotic syndrome are:
- Mesangiocapillary glomerulonephritis
- SLE
- IgA nephropathy.

Q.38. What are the mechanisms of nephritic syndrome?

Ans. Mechanisms of nephritic syndrome are:
- Inflammation
- Reactive cell proliferation
- Breaks in GBM
- Crescent formation.

Q.39. In AGN, is streptococcus directly infecting the kidney?

Ans. No, antibody formed against streptococcal antigen cross react with glomerular protein due to molecular mimicry.

Q.40. Which type of disease is this?

Ans. Immune-mediated.

Q.41. What are the mechanisms of nephrotic syndrome?

Ans. Mechanism of nephrotic syndrome are:
- Injury to podocytes
- Changed architecture—Scarring
- Deposition of matrix or other elements.

Q.42. What are the causes of rapidly progressive (crescentic) glomerulonephritis?

Ans. Causes are:
- Focal segmental (necrotizing) glomerulonephritis
- SLE
- Goodpasture's (anti-GBM) disease
- IgA nephropathy.

Q.43. What are the causes of glomerulonephritis associated with low serum complement?

Ans. Causes are:
- Postinfection glomerulonephritis, e.g. PSGN
- Subacute bacterial infection: Especially endocarditis
- SLE
- Cryoglobulinemia
- Mesangiocapillary glomerulonephritis, usually type II.

Q.44. A 5-year-old boy presented with puffiness of face with scanty micturition for last 3 days. What is your diagnosis?

Ans. Diagnosis is acute glomerulonephritis.

Q.45. What is the probable cause?

Ans. Poststreptococcal glomerulonephritis is the probable cause.

Q.46. What history would you take to detect underlying cause?

Ans. History of:
- Skin infection (infected scabies)
- Sore throat.

Q.47. What history will you take in case of AGN following scabies?

Ans. History of:
- Secondary infection of scabies
- Interval between infection and onset of AGN.

Q.48. What is the latency between infection and nephritis?

Ans. The latency is usually about 10 days after a throat infection or longer (2–3 weeks) after skin infection.

Q.49. If latency is 3 days, what would you think?

Ans. IgA nephropathy.

Q.50. What are the clinical features of AGN?

Ans. Symptoms—

- Swelling of the face followed by generalized swelling
- Scanty high colored urine (smoky)
- Sometimes history of sore throat/skin infections 2–3 weeks back.

Signs—

- Puffy face
- Pitting edema
- Hypertension
- Evidence of skin infection
- Signs of complications.

Q.51. How many adults with glomerulonephritis have hypertension?

Ans. 50% adult.

Q.52. What are the complications of AGN?

Ans. Complications are:

- Hypertensive encephalopathy
- Hypertensive LVF
- ARF
- Electrolyte imbalance.

Q.53. Suppose this patient develops severe breathlessness, what is your thinking?

Ans. Acute pulmonary edema due to hypertensive left ventricular failure.

Q.54. Suppose this patient becomes unconscious, what is your thinking?

Ans. Hypertensive encephalopathy.

Q.55. What are the investigations done in AGN?

Ans. Urine— R/M/E- RBC ++
Cast— RBC and granular cast)
Albumin +/++,

Blood— CBC with ESR

Serum urea and creatinine— May be raised
Serum electrolyte— K^+ may be raised
Serum C_3 level— Decreased
Bacteriological— Throat swab/swab from skin lesion for culture and sensitivity
ASO titer.

Q.56. What are the findings in routine examination of urine in AGN?

Ans. Urine— R/M/E-
RBC ++
Cast— RBC and granular cast
Albumin +/++
Dysmorphic RBC in phase contrast microscopy.

Q.57. What is the hallmark of glomerulonephritis?

Ans. Presence of dysmorphic RBC under phase contrast microscopy and/or RBC cast in urine.

Q.58. What is cast?

Ans. Casts are cylindrical structures (shape of renal tubule) composed mainly of mucoprotein (the Tamm-Horsefall mucoprotein) which is secreted by epithelial cells lining the loops of Henle, the distal tubules and the collecting ducts.

Common casts include—
Hyaline cast—Nephrotic syndrome
Granular cast—Urinary tract infection
RBC cast—Glomerulonephritis.

Q.59. What is treatment for AGN?

Ans. a. General measures
Bed rest—Increases GFR, so helps in reducing hypertension
Diet —Salt restricted diet
Protein restricted diet
Fluid (previous day urine output + 300 mL)
K^+ containing food restriction.

b. Supportive measures
- Edema—Diuretic, e.g. frusemide
- Antihypertensive drug—Calcium channel blocker e.g. amlodipine, ACE inhibitor
- Antibiotic—Phenoxymethylpenicillin/erythromycin for 10 days.

c. Treatment of complications if any.

d. Follow up:
- Pulse
- BP
- Edema

  - Weight
  - Maintain fluid intake output chart
  - Albumin chart.

Q.60. Which antihypertensives are preferred?

Ans. Preferred antihypertensives are:
- Calcium channel blocker, e.g. amlodipine
- ACE inhibitor if S.creatinine is less than 5 mg.

Q.61. Define nephrotic syndrome?

Ans. It is a clinical condition characterized by:
- Massive proteinuria: Usually > 3.5 gm/24 hours (urine may be frothy)
- Hypoalbuminemia (< 30 gm/L)
- Generalized edema
- Hyperlipidemia.

Q.62. What are the causes of nephrotic syndrome?

Ans. Causes of nephrotic syndrome are:
- Primary glomerular disease
  - Minimal change glomerular lesion
  - Focal segmental glomerular sclerosis
  - Membranous nephropathy
  - Membrano- proliferative GN
- Secondary glomerular disease
  - Systemic disease: Diabetes mellitus, amyloidosis, and SLE
  - Infections: HBV, HCV, HIV, malaria, and syphilis
  - Drugs and heavy metals
  - Malignancy: Lymphoma, Ca breast, Ca lung, and Ca colon.

Q.63. What are the common histological types of NS?

Ans. Common histological types of NS are:
- Minimal change glomerular lesion
- Focal segmental glomerular sclerosis
- Membranous nephropathy.

Q.64. What is minimal change lesion?

Ans. There is no abnormality on light microscopy but flatening of foot process under electron microscopy.

Q.65. What is the most common cause of nephrotic syndrome in children?

Ans. Minimal change nephropathy is the most common cause of nephrotic sysndrome in children.

Q.66. What is the most common cause of nephrotic syndrome in adults?

Ans. Membranous nephropathy is the most common cause of nephrotic syndrome in adults. Minimal change disease accounts for about one-quarter of nephrotic syndrome in adults.

Q.67. What is the presentation of nephrotic syndrome?

Ans. Swelling of the body usually starting from the face and then generalized edema-anasarca.

Q.68. What investigations will you do in nephrotic syndrome?

Ans. Urine—R/M/E (albumin +++/++++)
24 hour urinary protein (>3.5 gm/day)
Blood—CBC with ESR
Serum total protein—Decreased
Serum albumin— <30 gm/L
Serum cholesterol—Raised
Serum C_3 level —Normal
Renal function tests— Serum urea and creatinine
Serum electrolytes.
USG of KUB region
Investigation to find out secondary causes— RBS (DM)
ANA, anti dsDNA (SLE)
HBsAg (HBV)
Renal biopsy (confirmatory).

Q.69. What are the findings in blood investigations in case of nephrotic syndrome?

Ans. Blood—
- Serum total protein—Decreased
- Serum albumin— <30 gm/L
- Serum cholesterol—Raised
- Serum C_3 level—Normal
- Serum urea and creatinine—Raised if renal impairment
- Serum electrolytes.

Investigation to find out secondary causes—
- RBS (DM)
- ANA, anti dsDNA (SLE)
- HBsAg (HBV).

Q.70. What are the indications of renal biopsy in nephrotic syndrome?

Ans. Indications are:

- Nephrotic syndrome before 1 year
- Nephrotic syndrome after 8 years
- Serum C_3 level persistently declining for the past 3 months
- Steroid resistance
- Secondary cause of nephrotic syndrome.

Q.71. What are the indications of renal biopsy?

Ans. Indications are:

- Acute renal failure that is not adequately explained.
- Chronic renal failure with normal-sized kidneys.
- Nephrotic syndrome or glomerular proteinuria in adult.
- Nephrotic syndrome in children that has atypical features (hematuria, hypertension) or is not responding to treatment.
- Isolated hematuria with renal characteristics.
- Systemic diseases with renal involvement.

Q.72. What are the D/Ds of nephrotic syndrome?

Ans. D/Ds of nephrotic syndrome are:

- AGN
- Cirrhosis of the liver
- CCF
- PEM.

Q.73. What is the treatment for nephrotic syndrome?

Ans. i. General measures—

- Dietary sodium restriction.
- Fluid is not restricted.
- Diet: Balanced diet adequate in protein and calorie, not more than 30% calorie from fat.
- Edema—Thiazide, loop diuretics plus K^+ sparing diuretics is given.
- Hypercholesterolemia—Lipid lowering drugs (e.g. statins).
- Hypercoagulopathy—Anticoagulant (e.g. heparin).
- Infection—Antibiotics. Pneumococcal infections are particularly common and pneumococcal vaccine should be given.

ii. Specific measures—This depends on underlying histological type.

Minimal change nephropathy

Initial attack: Prednisolone 60 mg/m^2 body surface area daily (2–3 divided dose) for 6 weeks.

Then, 40 mg/m^2 body surface area single morning dose in alternate days for next 6 weeks.

Then, alternate day dose is slowly tapered and discontinued over next 2–3 months.

Relapse—Prednisolone 2 mg/kg/day till urine becomes negative for protein for 3 consecutive days. Then, 1.5 mg/kg/day single morning dose in alternate days for 4 weeks.

Frequent relapses—Treated by cyclophosphamide or cyclosporin.

Q.74. How can you follow up this patient?

Ans. Follow up of patient:

- Edema decreased or not (weight)
- Urine output
- Urinary albumin by bedside heat coagulation test
- Infection screening
- PUD (steroid induced)
- Appetite
- BP.

Q.75. What are the complications of nephrotic syndrome?

Ans. Complications of nephrotic syndrome are:

- Infection—Spontaneous peritonitis, pneumococcal sepsis, cellulitis, pneumonia, and UTI.
- Arterial and venous thrombosis
- Abdominal pain
- Hypovolemia
- Shock
- ARF
- Hypercholesterolemia
- PUD (steroid-induced)
- End stage renal disease.

Q.76. What is urinary remission in nephrotic syndrome?

Ans. Urine albumin nil or trace for consecutive 3 days is urinary remission in nephrotic syndrome.

Q.77. What is complete remission in nephrotic syndrome?

Ans. Protein-free urine along with serum albumin level >3.5 gm/dL is complete remission in nephrotic syndrome.

Q.78. What is relapse in nephrotic syndrome?

Ans. Urine albumin 3+ or 4+ for consecutive 3 days having been in remission previously.

Q.79. What is frequent relapse in nephrotic syndrome?

Ans. 2 or more relapses in 6 months of initial response or more than 3 relapses in 12 months is frequent relapse in nephrotic syndrome.

Q.80. What are infrequent relapses in nephrotic syndrome?

Ans. < 2 relapses in 6 months of initial response or less than 3 relapses in 12 months are imprequent relapses in nephrotic syndrome.

Q.81. What is steroid dependent in nephrotic syndrome?

Ans. 2 consecutive relapse when on alternate day steroids or within 14 days of discontinuation.

Q.82. What do you mean by steroid resistant in nephrotic syndrome?

Ans. Absence of remission despite therapy with 4 weeks of daily prednisolone dose of 2 mg/kg/day.

Q.83. What are the clinical types of nephrotic syndrome?

Ans. Clinical types of nephrotic syndrome are:
- Frequent relapse
- Infrequent relapse
- Steroid dependent
- Steroid resistant.

Q.84. Tell the prognosis of nephrotic syndrome.

Ans. Prognosis of nephrotic syndrome are:
- It depends on histological type.
- Minimal change disease—Prognosis is good, it does not progress to chronic kidney disease (CKD).
- Membranous nephropathy—Approximately one-third remit spontaneously, one-third remain in a nephrotic state, and one-third show progressive loss of renal function and progress to chronic kidney disease (CKD).
- FSGS—Poor, often progress to chronic kidney disease (CKD).

Q.85. Counselings in case of nephrotic syndrome.

Ans. Counselings are:

i. Counseling regarding disease
ii. Counseling regarding treatment

iii. Counseling regarding complications
iv. Counseling regarding prognosis.

Q.86. How can you differentiate between AGN and nephrotic syndrome?

Ans.

Traits	AGN	Nephrotic syndrome
Age	5–15 years usually	2–6 years usually
History: Pharyngitis or skin infection	Present	Absent
Clinical features:		
Hematuria	Present	Absent
Scratch mark	May be present	Absent
Hypertension	Present	May be present
Urine examination		
Color	High color	Normal
Protein	Mild to moderate	Massive
RBC and RBC cast	Present	Absent
Granular cast	Absent	Present
Serum C_3 level	Low	Normal
Relapse	Uncommon	Common
Treatment	Mainly supportive	Specific by prednisolone

Q.87. A 30-year-old man presents with loose motion and vomiting for 2 days. On query he admitted, he did not pass any urine for last 24 hours. What is your impression?

Ans. This patient develops acute renal failure (ARF) due to hypovolemia.

Q.88. What are the common causes of ARF?

Ans. Hypovolemia (decreased blood volume), usually from fluid loss (diarrhea), shock or excessive diuretics use.

Toxins or medication (e.g. some NSAIDs, aminoglycoside antibiotics) sepsis.

Q.89. How can you treat the patient of ARF following diarrhea?

Ans. Correction of dehydration by appropriate fluid (e.g. cholera saline).

Restoration of blood volume will restore kidney function and produce urine output.

If no urine output after rehydration, it indicates established ARF. So management of oliguric phase should be given—

- Hyperkalemia (a plasma K^+ concentration > 6 mmol/L) must be treated immediately, to prevent life-threatening cardiac arrhythmias.
- Fluid—Daily fluid intake should equal to urine output plus an additional 500 mL to cover insensible losses.
- Protein and energy intake— In patients in whom dialysis is likely to be avoided, accumulation of urea is slowed by dietary protein restriction (to about 40 gm/day).
- Infection control.
- Drugs—Vasoactive drugs such as NSAIDs and ACE inhibitors and nephrotoxic drugs should be avoided.
- Renal replacement therapy.

Q.90. What is acute renal failure?

Ans. Acute renal failure (ARF; also referred to as acute kidney injury, or AKI) describes a sudden and usually reversible loss of renal function, which develops over days or weeks and is usually accompanied by a reduction in urine volume.

Q.91. What is the RIFLE classification/consensus criteria of ARF?

Ans.

Grade	GFR criteria	UO criteria
Risk	SCr × 1.5 UO	< 0.5 mL/kg/hours × 6 hours
Injury	SCr × 2 UO	< 0.5 mL/kg/hours × 12 hours
Failure	SCr × 3 or SCr > 350 µmol/L with an acute rise > 40 µmol/L	< 0.3 mL/kg/hours × 24 hours UO < 0.3 mL/kg/ hours × 24 hours
Loss	Persistent ARF > 4 weeks	
ESKD	Persistent renal failure > 3 months	

Q.92. What is chronic renal failure (CRF)?

Ans. Chronic renal failure (CRF) refers to an irreversible deterioration in renal function which classically develops over a period of years.

Q.93. What are the causes of chronic kidney disease/chronic renal failure?

Ans. Causes of CKD/CRF are:

- Glomerulonephritis
- DM
- Hypertension
- Interstitial diseases
- Renal artery stenosis
- Systemic inflammatory diseases
- Polycystic kidney disease
- Unknown.

Q.94. What is the most common cause of CRF in developing countries?

Ans. Chronic glomerulonephritis is the most common cause of CRF in developing countries.

Q.95. What are the common causes of CKD worldwide?

Ans. Common causes of CKD worldwide are:

- Diabetes mellitus
- Hypertension
- Chronic glomerulonephritis.

Q.96. What are the stages of CKD?

Ans. Stages of chronic kidney disease (CKD)—

Stage	Description	GFR (mL/min/1.73 m^2)
1	Kidney damage with normal or ↑ GFR	≥ 90
2	Kidney damage with mild ↓ GFR	60–89
3	Moderate ↓ GFR	30–59
4	Severe ↓ GFR	15–29
5	Kidney failure	< 15 (or dialysis)

Q.97. What is difference between CKD and CRF?

Ans. CKD refers to all stages ranging from kidney damage with normal or raised GFR to kidney failure but CRF means at least some impairment of renal function.

Q.98. How does a patient of CKD usually present?

Ans. Patient of CKD usually present with—

- Asymptomatic—Detected on routine blood biochemistry, e.g. S. creatinine high.
- Anorexia, nausea, and vomiting.
- Weakness, lethargy, and pallor due to anemia.
- Later hiccup, pruritus, muscular twitching, fits, drowsiness, and coma.

Q.99. What are the stigmata of chronic kidney disease?

Ans. Stigmata of chronic kidney disease are:

- Pallor
- Pruritus
- Pigmentation
- Persistent hypertension
- Progressive back pain (renal osteodystrophy)
- Proximal myopathy
- Peripheral neuropathy.

Q.100. What are the common renal diseases causing hypertension?

Ans. The common renal diseases causing hypertension are:

- Glomerulonephritis
- Renovascular disease
- Interstitial diseases
- Renal artery stenosis
- Polycystic kidney disease.

Q.101. What are the causes of anemia in chronic renal failure?

Ans. Causes of anemia in chronic renal failure are:

- Relative deficiency of erythropoietin.
- Diminished erythropoiesis due to toxic effects of uremia on marrow precursor cells.
- Reduced red cell survival.
- Increased blood loss due to capillary fragility and poor platelet function.
- Reduced dietary intake and absorption and utilization of iron.

Q.102. How will you treat anemia in chronic renal failure?

Ans. Treatment of anemia in chronic renal failure are:

- First look for iron deficiency—Corrected by iron supplementation.
- Then, recombinant human erythropoietin—Target Hb level is 10–12 gm/dL.
- If severe anemia and blood transfusion.

Q.103. What are the components of renal osteodystrophy?

Ans. Components are:

- Osteomalacia
- Osteoporosis
- Osteosclerosis
- Hyperparathyroid bone disease (osteitis fibrosa cystica).

Q.104. What may be the findings of renal ultrasonography in chronic renal failure?

Ans. Renal ultrasound—

- Small echogenic kidneys with loss of corticomedullary differentiation are usual finding in advanced renal failure.
- Structural abnormalities, such as polycystic kidneys, also may be observed.
  - This is a useful test to screen for hydronephrosis.
  - Asymmetric renal size suggests renovascular or developmental disease.

Q.105. How will you treat chronic renal failure?

Ans.
1. Identify and treatment of the underlying renal disease
2. Renoprotection—

- Goals of treatment
  - BP < 120/80
  - Proteinuria < 0.3 gm/24 hours.

Treatment

- Patients with chronic kidney disease and proteinuria > 1 gm/24 hours:
- ACE inhibitor increasing to maximum dose.
- Add angiotensin receptor antagonist if goals are not achieved.
- Add diuretic to prevent hyperkalemia and help to control BP.

- Add calcium-channel blocker (verapamil or diltiazem) if goals not achieved.

Additional measures

- Statins to lower cholesterol to < 4.5 mmol/L
- Stop smoking (threefold higher rate of deterioration in CKD)
- Treat diabetes (HbA1c < 7%)
- Normal protein diet (0.8–1 gm/kg body weight).

3. Correction of complications

- Hyperkalemia—Limit K^+ intake to 70 mmol/day
- Acidosis—$NaHCO_3$
- Hypocalcemia and hyperphosphatemia—
  - Hypocalcemia—Vitamin D analogues
  - Hyperphosphatemia—Dietary restriction of high phosphate foods (milk, cheese, eggs), use of phosphate binding drugs with food such as $CaCO_3$ and $AL(OH)_3$, parathyroidectomy.

Drug therapy—

- This should be minimized in patients with chronic renal impairment.
- Tetracyclines (with the possible exception of doxycycline) should be avoided. Avoid nephrotoxic medications.
- Anemia—Ecombinant human erythropoietin, iron supplementation.
- Fluid and electrolyte balance—Fluid intake around 3 liters/day, Na^+ intake to 100 mmol/day.

4. Renal replacement therapy when indicated.

Q.106. What are the treatment modalities of hyperkalemia in case of CRF?

Ans. Treatment modalities are:

i. Pharmacological— 10% glucose and insulin
Salbutamol nebulization

ii. Dialysis

iii. Dietary potassium restriction.

Q.107. What do you mean by renal replacement therapy (RRT)?

Ans. Renal replacement therapy means the facility to replace functions of the kidney.

Q.108. What are the types of renal replacement therapy?

Ans. Types of renal replacement therapy are:

- Hemodialysis— Removal of toxic elements from the blood, which is filtered through a membrane while circulated outside of the body through a machine.
- Hemofiltration.
- Peritoneal dialysis—Filtration through the lining membrane of the abdominal cavity; fluid is instilled into the peritoneal cavity, then drained.
- Renal transplantation.

Q.109. What are the indications of renal replacement therapy?

Ans. Indications are:

- Hyperkalemia—Plasma potassium level is >6 mmol/L if not corrected by medical therapy.
- Fluid overload and pulmonary edema if not responding to diuretic therapy.
- Metabolic acidosis if medical therapy fails.
- Plasma urea level is >30 mmol/L.
- Plasma creatinine level is >600 µmol/L.
- Uremic pericarditis/ uremic encephalopathy.

Q.110. What is dialysis?

Ans. Dialysis is a process for removing waste materials and excess water from the blood, and is used primarily as an artificial replacement for lost kidney function in people with renal failure.

Q.111. What are the inherited causes of chronic kidney disease?

Ans. Inherited causes of chronic kidney disease are:

- Polycystic kidney disease
- Alport's syndrome.

Q.112. What are the mode of inheritance of polycystic kidney disease (PKD)?

Ans. Mode of inheritance are:

Adult polycystic kidney disease—Autosomal dominant

Infantile polycystic kidney disease—Autosomal recessive.

Q.113. What are the presentations of adult polycystic kidney disease?

Ans. Presentations are:

i. Vague discomfort in loin or abdomen due to increasing mass of renal tissue.
ii. Acute loin pain or renal colic due to hemorrhage into a cyst.
iii. Hypertension.
iv. Hematuria (with little or no proteinuria).
v. Urinary tract or cyst infections.
vi. Renal failure.

Q.114. Describe a typical renal colic.

Ans. A typical renal colic is an acute pain in the loin, which radiates round the flank to the groin and often into the testis or labium. The pain steadily increases in intensity to reach a peak in a few minutes. The patient is restless and generally tries unsuccessfully to obtain relief by changing position or pacing the room.

Q.115. What are the causes of renal colic?

Ans. Renal colic occurs due to ureteric obstruction most commonly due to calculi or 'stones', although a sloughed renal papilla, tumor or blood clot may be responsible.

Q.116. What are the types of urinary incontinence?

Ans. Types of urinary incontinence are:

i. Stress incontinence
ii. Urge incontinence
iii. Overflow incontinence
iv. Continual incontinence.

Q.117. What are the types of neurogenic bladder?

Ans. Types of neurogenic bladder are:

Atonic (lower motor neuron)
Hypertonic (upper motor neuron)
Cortical— Postcentral
Precentral
Frontal.

Q.118. What are the presentations of benign prostatic hypertrophy (BPH)?

Ans. Presentations are:

i. The primary symptoms of BPH (obstructive symptoms) are hesitancy, poor prolonged flow and a sensation of incomplete emptying.

ii. Secondary (irritative) symptoms are urinary frequency, urgency of micturition and urge incontinence.

Q.119. What is the treatment of BPH?

Ans. Treatment for benign prostatic hypertrophy are:

i. Medical
   Prostate < 40 cm^3:α-adrenoceptor blockers
   Prostate > 40 cm^3: 5 α-reductase inhibitors
ii. Nonsurgical intervention— Thermotherapy
iii. Surgical—
   Transurethral resection of prostate (TURP)
   Holmium laser enucleation
   Open prostatectomy.

Q.120. What are the common α-adrenoceptor blockers used to treat BPH?

Ans. Common α-adrenoceptor blockers used to treat BPH are:

- Tamsulosin
- Alfuzosin.

Q.121. What are the common 5α-reductase inhibitors used to treat BPH?

Ans. Common 5 α-reductase inhibitors used to treat BPH are:

- Finasteride
- Dutasteride.

CHAPTER 7

Diabetes Mellitus

Q.1. Definition of diabetes mellitus.

Ans. Diabetes mellitus is a metabolic disorder resulting in raised blood glucose from defects in insulin secretion, insulin action or both that arises from genetic as well as environmental factors.

Or

Diabetes mellitus is a clinical syndrome characterized by hyperglycemia caused by absolute or relative deficiency of insulin.

Q.2. What are the presentations of diabetes mellitus?

Ans. i. Asymptomatic—Detected on routine examination (e.g. for insurance purposes).

ii. Acute presentation with typical symptoms—Young people with classic triad of symptoms: Polyuria, thirst and weight loss.

iii. Subacute presentation with nonspecific symptoms—Lack of energy, visual blurring, pruritus vulvae or balanitis.

iv. With complications as the presenting feature, e.g. DKA With micro/macroangiopathy.

Q.3. What are the types of diabetes mellitus?

Ans. Types of diabetes mellitus:

Type 1 diabetes mellitus

Type 2 diabetes mellitus

Other specific types

Gestational diabetes mellitus.

Q.4. How can you differentiate between type I and type II diabetes mellitus?

Ans.

Features	Type I	Type II
Markers of β cell destruction	Present	Absent
Age of onset	<30 years	>30 years
Body habitus	Normal to wasted	Obese/overweight
Insulin reserve	Low/absent	Normal/high
Acute complication	DKA	HONK
Insulin therapy	Responsive	Responsive
Symptom	Sudden, classical	Gradual, atypical

Q.5. Can you tell WHO diagnostic criteria for diagnosis of diabetes mellitus?

Ans. WHO criteria for the diagnosis of diabetes are:

- Fasting plasma glucose > 7.0 mmol/L (126 mg/dL)
- Random plasma glucose > 11.1 mmol/L (200 mg/dL)
- One abnormal laboratory value is diagnostic in symptomatic individuals; two values are needed in asymptomatic people.

Q.6. What are the indications for oral glucose tolerance test?

Ans. Indications are:

- Fasting plasma glucose 6.1–7.0 mmol/L (110–126 mg/dL)
- Random plasma glucose 7.8–11.0 mmol/L (140–198 mg/dL).

Q.7. How to perform an oral glucose tolerance test (OGTT)?

Ans. Steps to perform an oral glucose tolerance test (OGTT) are:

- Preparation before the test.
- Unrestricted carbohydrate diet for 3 days.
- Fasted overnight for at least 8 hours.
- Rest for 30 minutes.
- Remain seated for the duration of the test with no smoking.

- Sampling.
- Plasma glucose is measured before and 2 hours after a 75 gm oral glucose drink.

Q.8. What is the values for fasting hyperglycemia and impaired glucose tolerance?

Ans. Fasting hyperglycemia 6.1–6.9 mmol/L (110–125 mg/dL) Impaired glucose tolerance 7.8–11.0 mmol/L (140–199 mg/dL).

Q.9. What are the symptoms of hyperglycemia?

Ans. The symptoms of hyperglycemia are:

- Thirst and dry mouth
- Polyuria
- Nocturia
- Tiredness, fatigue, and lethargy
- Noticeable change in weight (usually weight loss)
- Blurring of vision
- Pruritus vulvae and balanitis (genital candidiasis)
- Nausea and headache
- Hyperphagia; predilection for sweet foods
- Mood change, irritability, difficulty in concentrating, and apathy.

Q.10. What are the modalities of treatment in diabetes mellitus?

Ans. Modalities of treatment are:

- Diet
- Discipline
- Drugs—Oral hypoglycemic drugs (OHA)
  Insulin.

Q.11. Please outline the management of diabetes mellitus.

Ans. Type I—Insulin + Diet—

i. Obese—Low energy diet.
ii. Nonobese—Weight maintenance diet.

Type II—

i. Obese— Low energy diet+ exercise → metformin→ metformin+sulfonylurea → add glitazone/other → add insulin.
ii. Nonobese—Weight maintenance diet+ exercise→ sulfonylurea → sulfonylurea+metformin → add glitazone/other → add insulin.

Q.12. Please tell the guidelines for care of type II diabetes mellitus in Bangladesh.

Ans. Mild–Fasting glucose (FPG) <10.0 mmol/L = Diet and exercise.

Moderate—FPG >10.0- <14.0 mmol/L = Diet and exercise. Wait for 2–4 weeks, without improvement, start OHA.

Severe—FPG >14.0 mmol/L, initiate insulin.

Q.13. Please tell recommended composition of diet for people with diabetes.

Ans.

Dietary constituent	Percentage of energy intake
Carbohydrate	45–60%
Sucrose	Upto 10%
Fat (total)	< 35%
n–6 polyunsaturated	< 10%
n–3 polyunsaturated	Eat 1 portion (140 gm) oily fish once or twice weekly
Monounsaturated	10–20%
Saturated	< 10%
Protein	10–15% (do not exceed 1 gm/kg body weight)
Fruit/vegetables	5 portions daily

Q.14. What are the roles of exercise in management of diabetes mellitus?

Ans. It benefits in the following ways—

- Assists control of blood glucose, blood pressure, and lipids.
- Helps to reduce and maintain ideal body weight.
- Prevents atherosclerosis, CHD, CVD, and PVD.
- Improves insulin sensitivity, increase demand of blood supply of different vital tissues.

Q.15. Which type of exercise will do and how long?

Ans. Aerobic exercise, i.e. brisk walking, swimming, cycling, and jogging at least 30 minutes a day.

Q.16. Classify oral hypoglycemic agents?

Ans. i. Biguanide
- Metformin—It is used in overweight patient with diabetes mellitus

ii. Sulfonylureas
- Glimepiride
- Glipizide
- Tolbutamide
- Glibenclamide
- Glyburide (micronized)

iii. Nonsulfonylurea secretagogue (meglitinides)
- Repaglinide
- Nateglinide

iv. α-glucosidase inhibitor
- Acarbose
- Miglitol

v. Thiazolidinedione
- Rosiglitazone
- Pioglitazone

vi. DPP-IV (dipeptidyl peptidase-4) inhibitor(gliptin)
- Sitagliptin
- Vildagliptin
- Saxagliptin.

Q.17. What is the indication of metformin?

Ans. Overweight or obese patient with type II diabetes who fail to respond to dietary measures alone.

Q.18. What are the contraindications of metformin?

Ans. Impaired hepatic or renal function and alcohol intake are the contraindications of metformin.

Q.19. What is the complication?

Ans. Metformin can increase susceptibility to lactic acidosis.

Q.20. What is the indication of sulfonylurea?

Ans. In the treatment of nonobese patients with type II diabetes who fail to respond to dietary measures alone.

Q.21. What is the mechanism of action of DPP-4 inhibitors?

Ans. DPP-4 inhibitors inhibit the enzyme, dipeptidyl peptidase 4 which rapidly degradate glucagon-like peptide (GLP-1).

Q.22. What is glucagon-like peptide (GLP-1)?

Ans. Glucagon-like peptide (GLP-1) is an incretin hormone (gut hormone).

Q.23. What are the actions of glucagon-like peptide (GLP-1)?

Ans.
- i. GLP-1 stimulates insulin secretion in a glucose-dependent manner and thus control hyperglycemia but does not cause hypoglycemia.
- ii. GLP-1 suppresses glucagon secretion.
- iii. It delays gastric emptying.
- iv. It reduces appetite.
- v. It encourages weight loss.

Q.24. What are the indications (uses) of insulin therapy?

Ans. Indications of insulin therapy are:
- i. All the patients of type 1 diabetes mellitus.
- ii. Pregnancy with diabetes mellitus.
- iii. Acute metabolic decompensated states in type II diabetes mellitus (DKA, HONK, lactic acidosis).
- iv. Type II diabetes mellitus with OHA failure.
- v. Acute stressful condition (infection, trauma, myocardial infarction).
- vi. During major surgery.
- vii. Advanced complication of diabetes mellitus (nephropathy and retinopathy).

Q.25. What are the insulin preparations?

Ans.

Insulin	Onset(hr)	Duration(hr)
Rapid-acting (insulin analogues: Lispro, aspart, glulisine)	< 0.5	3–4.5
Short-acting soluble (regular)	0.5–1	4–8
Intermediate-acting (isophane (NPH), lente)	1–3	7–14
Long-acting (bovine ultralente)	2–4	12–30
Long-acting (insulin analogues: glargine, detemir)	1–2	18–24

Q.26. What are the side effects of insulin?

Ans. Side effects of insulin are:

- Hypoglycemia
- Weight gain
- Allergy
- Insulin edema
- Lipodystrophy.

Q.27. Can you demonstrate how to inject insulin subcutaneously?

Ans. Steps to inject insulin subcutaneously are:

- Needle sited at right angle to the skin.
- Subcutaneous (not intramuscular) injection.
- Delivery devices: Glass syringe (requires resterilization), plastic syringe (disposable), pen device, infusion pump.

Q.28. What are the commonly used sites for insulin injection?

Ans. Main areas used are:

- Anterior abdominal wall
- Upper thighs/buttocks
- Upper outer arms.

Q.29. What are the routes of administration of insulin?

Ans. Routes of administration are:

- Subcutaneous
- IV (in DKA)
- IM (in DKA).

Q.30. What are the targets of treatment in diabetic patient?

Ans. Targets of treatment are:

i. Targets of glycemic control:
   - HbA1c <7.0%
   - Fasting blood glucose<6.1 mmol/L
   - Postprandial BG <8.0 mmol/L
   - Bed time BG<7.0 mmol/L.

ii. Targets of BP in diabetic person:
   - BP<130/80 mmHg
   - BP<120/70 mmHg in renal diseases.

iii. Targets of blood lipids in diabetic person:
   - LDL cholesterol<100 mg/dL
   - HDL cholesterol> 40 mg/dL
   - Triglyceride< 150 mg/dL.

Q.31. What is HbA1c?

Ans. HbA1c is glycosylated hemoglobin which provides an accurate and objective measure of glycemic control over a period of weeks to months (3 month).

Q.32. What are the complications of diabetes mellitus?

Ans. Acute complications

- DKA (diabetic ketoacidosis)
- HONK (hyperosmolar nonketotic diabetic coma)
- Lactic acidosis
- Hypoglycemia.

Chronic complications

- Microvascular complications:
  - Diabetic retinopathy
  - Diabetic nephropathy
  - Diabetic neuropathy
- Macrovascular complications:
  - Coronary artery diseases
  - Cerebrovascular diseases
  - Peripheral artery diseases.

Q.33. A 50-year-old diabetic man on insulin went to walk in the morning after taking insulin. He was found unconscious. What may be the possibilities?

Ans. Possibilities are:

- Hypoglycemia
- Other causes of coma.

Q.34. How can you manage the patient?

Ans. Management—

- Immediate assessment by checking vital signs.
- Maintenance of ABC.
- Short history from available source, e.g. not taking breakfast.
- IV access and blood sample for blood sugar and other tests.
- IV glucose—100 mL of 25% glucose stat followed by 10% dextrose 1000 cc.

Q.35. What is hypoglycemia?

Ans. When blood glucose is < 3.5 mmol/L (63 mg/dL) in a diabetic patient (<2.2 mmol/L in normal person), it is called hypoglycemia.

Q.36. What is severe hypoglycemia?

Ans. When external help is required to recover, it is called severe hypoglycemia.

Q.37. What are the features of hypoglycemia?

Ans. Most common symptoms of hypoglycemia are:

Autonomic
- Sweating
- Trembling
- Pounding heart
- Hunger
- Anxiety.

Neuroglycopenic
- Confusion
- Drowsiness
- Speech difficulty
- Inability to concentrate
- Incoordination
- Irritability and anger.

Nonspecific
- Nausea
- Tiredness
- Headache.

Q.38. What are the common causes of hypoglycemia?

Ans. Common causes of hypoglycemia are:
- Missed, delayed or inadequate meal
- Unexpected or unusual exercise
- Alcohol
- Errors in oral antidiabetic agent(s) or insulin dose/schedule/administration.

Q.39. How can you differentiate hypoglycemic coma and DKA at bed side?

Ans.

Traits	Hypoglycemic coma	DKA
History	No food Vigorous exercise Insulin overdose	Little or no insulin Infection
Onset	In good previous health, related to last insulin injection	Ill health for several days

Contd...

Contd...

Traits	Hypoglycemic coma	DKA
Symptoms	Palpitation, sweating, hunger	Polyuria, thirst, abdominal pain and vomiting
Signs	Moist skin and tongue Full pulse Normal or raised systolic BP Shallow or normal breathing Brisk reflexes No smell of acetone	Dry skin and tongue Weak pulse Low BP Air hunger Diminished reflexes Smell of acetone

Q.40. Suppose you cannot differentiate at bed side, which treatment would you start?

Ans. IV glucose as hypoglycemic coma is more dangerous.

Q.41. What are the causes of hyperglycemic coma?

Ans. Causes are:

- DKA (diabetic ketoacidosis)
- HONK (hyperosmolar nonketotic diabetic coma).

Q.42. How can you differentiate at bed side?

Ans.

DKA	HONK
Commonly occurs in type I diabetes mellitus, but may occur in type II	Occurs in type II diabetes mellitus
Common in children and young	Common in elderly
Dehydration less severe	Dehydration more severe
More breathless, air hunger	Little or no breathless
Acetone breath	No smell of acetone

Q.43. What are the causes of DKA?

Ans. Causes are:

- Undiagnosed diabetes mellitus
- Omission of insulin dose
- Injudicious reduction of insulin dose

- Intercurrent illness specially acute infection
- Trauma
- Pregnancy.

Q.44. What are the cardinal biochemical features of DKA?

Ans. Cardinal biochemical features are:
- Hyperglycemia
- Hyperketonemia
- Metabolic acidosis.

Q.45. What are the clinical features of DKA?

Ans. Symptoms
- Polyuria and thirst
- Weakness
- Nausea and vomiting
- Abdominal pain
- Impairment of level of consciousness.

Signs
- Dehydration
- Hypotension (postural or supine)
- Tachycardia
- Air hunger (Kussmaul breathing)
- Smell of acetone.

Q.46. What are the principles of management of DKA?

Ans.
i. The administration of short-acting (soluble) insulin
ii. Fluid replacement
iii. Potassium replacement
iv. Administration of antibiotics if infection is present.

Q.47. What is the average loss of fluid and electrolytes in adult diabetic ketoacidosis of moderate severity?

Ans. Water: 6 L
Sodium: 500 mmol
Chloride: 400 mmol
Potassium: 350 mmol
3 L extracellular replaced with saline, 3 L intracellular replaced with dextrose.

Q.48. What are the principles of management of HONK?

Ans. Principles of management are:
i. The administration of short-acting (soluble) insulin.
ii. Fluid replacement.
iii. Administration of antibiotics if infection is present.

iv. Prophylactic low molecular weight heparin to prevent thromboembolic complication.

Q.49. What are the differences in the treatment of HONK from treatment of DKA?

Ans. Differences are:

i. Insulin requirement is less in HONK than in DKA.
ii. Fluid replacement is done by 0.45% NaCl in HONK in contrast to 0.9% NaCl in DKA.
iii. No need of potassium replacement.

Q.50. What are the types of retinopathy?

Ans. Types of retinopathy are:

- Nonproliferative 'background' retinopathy without maculopathy.
- Maculopathy.
- Preproliferative retinopathy.
- Proliferative retinopathy.

Q.51. How can you differentiate between diabetic and hypertensive retinopathy?

Ans.

Character	Diabetic retinopathy	Hypertensive retinopathy
Arteriolar thickening, tortuosity and increased reflectiveness (silver wiring)	Absent	Present
Arteriovenous nipping	Absent	Present in grade 2
Hemorrhages	Dot and blot	Flame-shaped
Exudates	Soft	Hard
Papilledema	Absent	Present in grade 4
Neovascularization	Present in proliferative retinopathy	Absent

Q.52. Classify diabetic neuropathy.

Ans. i. Somatic

Polyneuropathy

- Symmetrical, mainly sensory and distal.
- Asymmetrical, mainly motor and proximal (including amyotrophy).

Mononeuropathy (including mononeuritis multiplex).

ii. Autonomic.

Q.53. What do you mean by microalbuminuria? What is it significance in diabetic patient?

Ans. Microalbuminuria means the urinary excretion of small amounts of albumin (20–200 µg/min or 30–300 mg/24 hours).

The presence of microalbuminuria is a clear sign of glomerular abnormality and can detect the very early stages of progressive glomerular disease, i.e. diabetic nephropathy.

Q.54. What is the natural history of diabetic nephropathy?

Ans. Stage of hyperfiltration → microalbuminuria → sustained proteinuria → nephrotic range proteinuria → end stage renal disease.

Q.55. What is gestational diabetes mellitus?

Ans. Hyperglycemia occurring for the first time during pregnancy is termed gestational diabetes.

Q.56. What are the causes of glycosuria?

Ans. Causes are:

i. Diabetes mellitus
ii. Alimentary glycosuria—In normal people or after gastric surgery, hyperthyroidism, peptic ulceration or hepatic disease.
iii. Pregnancy.

Q. 57. Name one condition where renal threshold is decreased.

Ans. In pregnancy renal threshold is decreased.

CHAPTER 8

Endocrine System

Q.1. Name some endocrine diseases.

Ans. Some endocrine diseases are hypothyroidism, thyrotoxicosis, diabetes mellitus, hyperparathyroidism, hypogonadism, adrenal insufficiency, and Cushing's syndrome.

Q.2. What are the major endocrine glands?

Ans. Pituitary gland, thyroid gland, parathyroid gland, endocrine pancreas, adrenal gland, and testes or ovary are the major endocrine glands.

Q.3. Name some hyperactive and hypoactive diseases in endocrine system.

Ans.

Gland	Hyperactive	Hypoactive
Pituitary	Acromegaly	Dwarfism
Thyroid	Thyrotoxicosis	Hypothyroidism
Parathyroid	Hyperparathyroidism	Hypoparathyroidism
Adrenal	Cushing's syndrome	Addison's disease

Q.4. A middle-aged women presented with constipation, hoarseness of voice and cold intolerance. What is your probable diagnosis?

Ans. Probable diagnosis is hypothyroidism.

Q.5. Define hypothyroidism?

Ans. It is a clinical condition resulting from reduced circulatory level of thyroid hormone.

Q.6. What are the common causes of primary hypothyroidism?

Ans. Common causes of primary hypothyroidism are:
- Spontaneous atrophic hypothyroidism.
- Radioactive iodine ablation.
- Thyroidectomy.
- Hashimoto's thyroiditis.

Q.7. What is the most common cause of primary hypothyroidism?

Ans. The most common cause of primary hypothyroidism is iodine deficiency, e.g. in mountainous regions.

Q.8. What are the common causes of transient hypothyroidism?

Ans. The common causes of transient hypothyroidism are:
- Subacute thyroiditis
- Postpartum thyroiditis.

Q.9. What do you mean by primary hypothyroidism?

Ans. Primary hypothyroidism means disease in the thyroid gland.

Q.10. What do you mean by secondary hypothyroidism?

Ans. Secondary hypothyroidism means disease in the pituitary gland or hypothalamus.

Q.11. How can you differentiate primary and secondary hypothyroidism?

Ans.

Points	Primary	Secondary hypothyroidism
Clinically	Weight gain myxedematous	Weight loss Lean and thin
Biochemically	TSH raised	TSH low

Q.12. What are the common presentations of hypothyroidism?

Ans. Common presentations are:
- Unusual tiredness
- Swelling of the body (nonpitting edema)
- Weight gain
- Cold intolerance
- Hoarseness of voice
- Constipation.

Q.13. What questions will you ask if you suspect hypothyroidism?

Ans. Do you notice any change in your weight? (weight gain)
Do you notice any change in your voice? (hoarseness of voice)
Do you prefer hot or cold? (cold intolerance)
What is your bowel habit? (constipation)
What is your menstrual history (in female)? (menorrhagia).

Q.14. What are the common findings on examination?

Ans. Common findings are:

- Hoarseness of voice
- Dry scaly skin
- Puffy face with periorbital edema
- Sinus bradycardia
- Nonpitting edema
- Delayed relaxation of ankle jerk.

Q.15. One disease can be diagnosed by over telephone, which is the disease?

Ans. The disease is hypothyroidism.

Q.16. Ask one question to a patient of hypothyroidism and what 2 clues can you get from the patient's answer?

Ans. Ask the patient about weight change, so when he/she answers you will know if he/she is having weight gain or weight loss and you will also know if he/she has a husky voice.

Q.17. Which biochemical investigations would you suggest to diagnose hypothyroidism?

Ans. Biochemical investigations are serum T_4 and TSH.

Q.18. Why not serum T_3?

Ans. Measurements of serum T_3 are unhelpful since they do not discriminate reliably between euthyroidism and hypothyroidism.

Q.19. What are the expected findings in primary hypothyroidism?

Ans. The expected findings in primary hypothyroidism are serum T_4 low and TSH raised.

Q.20. What are the expected findings in secondary hypothyroidism?

Ans. The expected findings in secondary hypothyroidism are serum T_4 low and TSH also low.

Q.21. If single investigation is asked for hypothyroidism, which one?

Ans. TSH.

Q.22. How to interpret thyroid function test results.

Ans.

TSH	T_4	T_3	Most likely interpretation(s)
Undetectable	Raised	Raised	Primary thyrotoxicosis
Undetectable	Normal	Raised	Primary T_3-toxicosis
Undetectable	Normal	Normal	Subclinical thyrotoxicosis
Elevated > 20 mU/L	Low	Low	Primary hypothyroidism
Undetectable/ normal	Low	Low	Secondary hypothyroidism
Mildly elevated 5–20 mU/L	Low	Low	Primary hypothyroidism Secondary hypothyroidism
Mildly elevated 5–20 mU/L	Normal	Normal	Subclinical hypothyroidism
Elevated	Raised	Raised	Noncompliance with T_4 replacement-recent 'loading' dose Secondary thyrotoxicosis

Q.23. What are the ECG findings in hypothyroidism?

Ans. Sinus bradycardia with low voltage ECG.

Q.24. How will you treat the patient?

Ans. Treat the patient by lifelong thyroxine therapy.

Q.25. What is the protocol of giving thyroxine?

Ans. 50 µg (one tablet) daily for 3 weeks (given in morning in empty stomach) 100 µg daily for 3 weeks.

Then maintenance dose at 100–150 µg daily 6 weeks should pass before repeating TFTs following a dose change.

It is necessary to measure thyroid function every 1–2 years, once dose of thyroxine is stabilized.

Q.26. What is the aim of treatment?

Ans. To maintain serum TSH within the normal reference range is the aim of treatment.

Q.27. In which conditions initial small dose (25 μg) is used?

Ans. Conditions are:

- Patient with IHD
- Elderly patient.

Q.28. Tell the treatment of hypothyroidism in pregnancy.

Ans. The dose of thyroxine should be increased usually by 50 μg of thyroxine.

Q.29. What will happen if inadequate replacement is given during pregnancy?

Ans. Inadequate maternal thyroxine replacement may result in congenital hypothyroidism of the baby.

Q.30. What is myxedema coma?

Ans. This is a rare presentation of hypothyroidism in which there is a depressed level of consciousness, usually in an elderly patient who appears myxedematous.

Q.31. What is myxdema madness?

Ans. Psychotic condition developed in a patient with hypothyroidism.

Q.32. Tell the follow up of hypothyroid patient after treatment.

Ans.
i. Clinical: Check for weight loss and decreased edema every two weeks till patient becomes euthyroid.
ii. Biochemical: TSH is checked every 3–6 weeks until patient is euthyroid.
   - After that monthly follow up for 3 months.
   - Then every 3–6 months follow up.

Q.33. What are the clinical criteria of remission of hypothyroidism?

Ans. Clinical criteria are:

- Reduction of weight
- Decreased edema
- Relief of constipation
- Husky voice takes about 3–6 months to normalize.

Q.34. What are the causes of hyperthyroidism?

Ans. Causes of hyperthyroidism are:

- Graves disease (60%–80%)
- Toxic multinodular goiter (14%)
- Toxic solitary nodule (5%)
- Thyroiditis, e.g. subacute (de Quervain's), postpartum.
- Iodide-induced—Drugs (e.g. amiodarone), radiographic contrast media.

Q.35. What are the common causes of hyperthyroidism?

Ans. Common causes of hyperthyroidism are:

- Graves disease (60%–80%)
- Toxic multinodular goiter (14%)
- Toxic solitary nodule (5%).

Q.36. What is the most common cause of hyperthyroidism?

Ans. The most common cause is Graves disease.

Q.37. What do you mean by thyrotoxicosis?

Ans. It is defined as a state of thyroid hormone excess.

Q.38. What do you mean by hyperthyroidism?

Ans. It is defined as a state which results in excessive thyroid function.

Q.39. What is primary and secondary hyperthyroidism?

Ans.

- Primary hyperthyroidism (thyrotoxicosis) is due to disease of thyroid gland.
- Secondary hyperthyroidism (thyrotoxicosis) is secondary to pituitary or hypothalamic disease.

Q.40. What are the causes of thyrotoxicosis without hyperthyroidism?

Ans. Subacute thyroiditis

Postpartum thyroiditis

Other—Thyroid destruction: Amiodarone, radiation, infarction or adenoma.

Thyrotoxicosis factitious (self-induced—thyroxine administration).

Q.41. What are the common causes of transient hyperthyroidism?

Ans. The common causes are:

- Subacute thyroiditis
- Postpartum thyroiditis.

Q.42. What are the common causes of thyrotoxicosis with less or normal iodine uptake?

Ans. Common causes are:

- Subacute thyroiditis
- Postpartum thyroiditis
- Drug-induced— amiodarone
- Radiation thyroiditis.

Q.43. What are the clinical triad of Graves disease?

Ans. Clinical triad are:

- Diffuse goiter
- Exophthalmos
- Pretibial myxedema.

Q.44. What are the common presentations of hyperthyroidism?

Ans. Common presentations are:

- Weight loss despite normal or increased appetite.
- Heat intolerance
- Excessive sweating
- Tremor
- Palpitation
- Diarrhea
- Hyperdefecation
- Proptosis.

Q.45. What are the causes of significant weight loss despite good appetite?

Ans. Causes are:

- Thyrotoxicosis
- Diabetes mellitus.

Q.46. Please tell the pathogenesis of weight loss in hyperthyroid.

Ans. Weight loss is due to the increased metabolic rate.

Q.47. What questions will you ask if you suspect hyperthyroidism?

Ans. Questions are:

- Do you notice any change in your weight? (weight loss)
- What is your appetite? (increased appetite)
- Do you prefer hot or cold? (heat intolerance)
- What is your bowel habit? (diarrhea)

- What is your menstrual history (in female)? (scanty mense).

Q.48. What are the common findings on examination?

Ans. Common findings are:

- Anxious looking
- Tremor on outstressed hands
- Warm sweaty hands
- Sinus tachycardia or atrial fibrillation
- Proptosis, lid lag, lid retraction
- Goiter +/– bruit
- Pretibial myxedema
- Proximal myopathy.

Q.49. What are the causes of tachycardia in hyperthyroidism?

Ans. Causes are:

- Sinus tachycardia
- Atrial fibrillation.

Q.50. What are the signs will you find in thyrotoxicosis in hand/ neck/ eye?

Ans. In hands—

i. Tremor on outstressed hands
ii. Warm sweaty hands
iii. Sinus tachycardia or atrial fibrillation or ectopics in radial pulse
iv. Clubing and onycholysis in Graves thyrotoxicosis.

In neck—

i. Goiter—Difuse goiter, multiple nodules or solitary nodule.
ii. Bruit in Graves' disease.

In eyes—Lid lag, lid retraction, proptosis, chemosis, and external ophthalmoplegia.

Q.51. What are the investigations done in hyperthyroidism?

Ans. i. To detect thyrotoxicosis

Serum T_3, T_4, and TSH

- Primary thyrotoxicosis—Increased T_3 and T_4, and decreased or undetectable TSH.
- Primary T_3 thyrotoxicosis—Increased T_3, normal T_4, and TSH undetectable.
- Subclinical thyrotoxicosis—T_3 and T_4 in the upper part of normal range and TSH undetectable.

ii. To establish the cause

a. TSH receptor antibody: Elevated in Graves disease.
b. Antiperoxidase and antithyroglobulin antibody: Very high in Hashimoto's thyroiditis, but slight to moderate high in Graves disease.
c. Isotope scanning.
d. USG of thyroid gland.

Q.52. If single investigation is asked for hyperthyroidism, which one?

Ans. Free T_4.

Q.53. What are the modalities of treatment of hyperthyroidism?

Ans. Modalities of treatment are:
- Antithyroid drugs
- Subtotal thyroidectomy
- Radioactive iodine therapy.

Q.54. Name antithyroid drugs.

Ans. Antithyroid drugs are:
- Carbimazole/methimazole
- Propylthiouracil.

Q.55. What are the side effects of antithyroid drugs?

Ans. Side effects are:
- Agranulocytosis
- Rashes.

Q.56. What is agranulocytosis?

Ans. A marked decrease in granulocytes, more commonly neutrophils. In agranulocytosis, the concentration of granulocytes (neutrophils, basophils, and eosinophils) drops below 100 cells/mm^3 of blood, which is less than 5% of the normal value.

Q.57. What advice would you give to the patient on antithyroid drugs?

Ans. To seek immediate medical attention if they develop unexplained fever or sore throat.

Q.58. What are the contraindications of radioactive iodine therapy?

Ans. Contraindications are:
- Pregnancy and breastfeeding
- Planned pregnancy within 6 months
- Active Graves ophthalmopathy.

Q.59. What are the complications of radioactive iodine?

Ans. Complications are:

i. The majority of patients eventually develop hypothyroidism.
ii. It may precipitate thyrotoxic crisis.
iii. Radiation thyroiditis.
iv. It may worsen ophthalmopathy.

Q.60. What is the role of β-blocker in the treatment of thyrotoxicosis?

Ans. β-blocker (propranolol 160 mg daily) causes symptomatic improvement by reducing sympathetic nervous symptoms such as tremor, tachycardia, and sweating.

Q.61. How can you follow up the patient?

Ans. Follow up:

i. Clinical: Check for weight and pulse rate
ii. Biochemical: Free T_3 and free T_4.

Q.62. How will you treat thyrotoxicosis in pregnancy?

Ans. i. Antithyroid drug—Propylthiouracil (150 mg /day) is the drug of choice.
NB: Carbimazole can cross placental barrier and can cause skin defect in the baby known as aplasia cutis.

ii. Subtotal thyroidectomy—It is performed if there is poor drug compliance or drug hypersensitivity. The surgery is most safely performed in 2nd trimester.
NB: Radioactive iodine is absolutely contraindicated as it induces fetal hypothyroidism.

Q.63. Tell the complications of thyrotoxicosis with their management?

Ans. i. Atrial fibrillation
Management:
a. β-blocker propranolol (verapamil/amiodarone if contraindicated).
b. Antithyroid drugs
c. Anticoagulation with warfarin.

ii. Heart failure
Management: Diuretics
Digoxin
Stop β-blocker.

iii. Ophthalmopathy
Management:
a. Cessation of smoking
b. Artificial tear drop
c. Oral prednisolone if severe inflammation
d. Urgent surgical decompression if visual acuity loss.

iv. Dermopathy (pretibial myxedema)
Management: Local steroids.

Q.64. A 40-year-old male presents with progressively worsening headache and sweating for 6 months. On query he admitted history of clash with door and bystander, increasing size of shoes and ring. What is your diagnosis?

Ans. Acromegaly is the diagnosis.

Q.65. What is acromegaly?

Ans. It is a clinical condition characterized by hypersecretion of growth hormone after closure of bony epiphysis (acro means periphery, megaly means large).

Q.66. What happens if it occurs before closure of epiphysis?

Ans. Gigantism.

Q.67. What is the cause for acromegaly?

Ans. Pituitary macroadenoma is the cause for acromegaly.

Q.68. What investigations will you do in acromegaly?

Ans. Investigations are:
- Measurement of growth hormone during OGTT
- X-ray skull lateral view (enlarged sella tursica)
- CT/MRI of brain
- IGF-1 (increased).

Q.69. What is the management of acromegaly?

Ans. **1st line therapy**
- Surgery—Transsphenoidal (microadenoma).

2nd line therapy
- Radiotherapy.

3rd line therapy
- Medical R_x (aim: to reduce growth hormone levels below 5 mu/L).
  - 1st somatostatin analogue—Octreotide/lanreotide
  - Growth hormone receptor antagonist—Pegvisomant

Newer therapy—Stereotectic surgery.

Q.70. What is Cushing's syndrome?

Ans. Cushing's syndrome is a clinical condition caused by excessive activation of glucocorticoid receptors.

Q.71. What is the most common cause of Cushing's syndrome?

Ans. Iatrogenic, due to prolonged administration of synthetic glucocorticoids such as prednisolone.

Q.72. What are the causes of Cushing's syndrome?

Ans. Causes are:

ACTH dependent
- Pituitary adenoma secreting ACTH (Cushing's disease)
- Ectopic ACTH syndrome (small-cell lung carcinoma)
- Iatrogenic (ACTH therapy).

Non-ACTH dependent
- Iatrogenic (chronic glucocorticoid therapy)
- Adrenal adenoma
- Adrenal carcinoma.

Pseudo-Cushing's syndrome
- Alcohol excess
- Major depressive illness
- Primary obesity.

Q.73. What is Cushing's disease?

Ans. Cushing's syndrome due to pituitary cause, e.g. pituitary adenoma.

Q.74. What are the common clinical features of Cushing's syndrome?

Ans. Common clinical features are:
- Central obesity
- Moon face
- Plethoric face
- Buffalo hump
- Hirsutism
- Acne
- Thin skin/easy bruising, purpura
- Striae (purple or red)
- Hypertension
- Hyperglycemia
- Osteoporosis
- Proximal myopathy.

Q.75. What are the investigations done in Cushing's syndrome?

Ans. a. To establish presence of Cushing's syndrome:
   i. Screening tests–
      - Overnight dexamethasone suppression test
      - 24 hours urinary free cortisol
   ii. Confirmatory–
      - Low dose dexamethasone suppression test (0.5 mg every 6 hours for 48 hours).
      - Circadian plasma cortisol.

b. To determine the underlying cause:
   Plasma ACTH levels—
   i. If high ACTH levels—
      - High-dose dexamethasone suppression test (2 mg every 6 hours for 2 days).
      - CRH infusion tests/Inferior petrosal sinus sampling.
      - Pituitary MRI scan with gadolinium contrast.
      - High-resolution chest CT—Ectopic ACTH production.
   ii. If ACTH levels undetectable
      CT scan of the abdomen—Adrenal tumors and bilateral hyperplasia.

c. To see complications:
   - Serum electrolytes
   - RBS and glycosylated Hb
   - Bone mineral density (BMD)
   - Lipid profile.

Q.76. What is the treatment of Cushing's syndrome?

Ans. Treatment—
   i. General
      - Prophylaxis against osteoporosis
      - PPI
      - Treatment of hyperlipidemia
      - Treatment of hypertension
      - Treatment of diabetes mellitus.
   ii. Specific
      a. Iatrogenic—Gradual withdrawal of steroid if possible.
      b. Cushing's disease—Transsphenoidal surgery with selective removal of the adenoma.

If unsuccessful bilateral adrenalectomy.

c. Adrenal tumors—Adrenal adenoma—Resection via laparoscopy or a loin incision.
d. Adrenal carcinomas—Resection if possible, tumor bed irradiation and adrenolytic drug such as mitotane.
e. Ectopic ACTH syndrome—Localization and removal of the tumor if possible.
   In case of nonresectable malignancies, medical therapy.

Q.77. What is Nelson's syndrome?

Ans. Nelson's syndrome is increased pigmentation (because of high levels of ACTH) associated with an enlarging pituitary tumor, which occurs in about 20% of cases after bilateral adrenalectomy for Cushing's disease.

Q.78. A patient with bronchial asthma was under good control with medication. He went to see his daughter far away from his house but forgot to bring his medicines. Without medication he was free from breathless but in the next morning he developed nausea, vomiting, and collapsed. What is your diagnosis?

Ans. Adrenal crisis is the diagnosis.

Q.79. How can you manage adrenal crisis?

Ans. Management—

i. Correction of volume depletion IV normal saline as required to normalize BP and pulse.
ii. Replacement of glucocorticoids IV hydrocortisone succinate 100 mg stat and hydrocortisone (50–100 mg IM 6-hourly) until the patient is well enough for reliable oral therapy.
iii. Correction of hypoglycemia. IV 10% glucose.

Q.80. What history would you take?

Ans. History of taking steroid.

Q.81. What is the most common cause of adrenal insufficiency?

Ans. Withdrawal of suppressive glucocorticoid therapy.

Q.82. What do you mean by adrenal insufficiency?

Ans. Adrenal insufficiency results from inadequate secretion of cortisol and/or aldosterone. It is potentially fatal and notoriously variable in its presentation.

Q.83. What is Addison's disease?

Ans. Addison's disease is the primary adrenal insufficiency.

Q.84. What are the presentations of Addison's disease?

Ans. Presentations are:

- Chronic presentation
- Acute presentation (adrenal crisis)
- Acute on chronic presentation.

Q.85. What are the common features of chronic presentation?

Ans. WPP—W-weakness, P-pigmentation, and P-postural hypotension are the common features of chronic presentation.

Q.86. What are the common causes of Addison's disease?

Ans. Common causes are:

- Autoimmune
- Tuberculosis
- HIV/AIDS
- Metastatic carcinoma
- Bilateral adrenalectomy.

Q.87. What are the sites commonly search for pigmentation?

Ans. Sites are:

- Buccal mucosa
- Sun-exposed areas—Face
- Pressure areas, (e.g. elbows, knees)
- Palmar creases, knuckles
- Recent scars.

Q.88. What are the investigations done in Addison's disease?

Ans. Investigations are:

i. Assessment of glucocorticoids
   - ACTH stimulation test

ii. Assessment of mineralocorticoids
   - Plasma electrolyte measurements—Hyponatremia and hyperkalemia.

iii. Other tests to establish the cause and association
   - Thyroid function tests.
   - Full blood count.
   - Plasma calcium and glucose.
   - Chest X-ray.
   - Test for gonadal function.
   - CT/MRI to identify malignancy.

Q.89. What is the finding of chest X-ray in Addison's disease?

Ans. Small heart (microcardia) is the findings.

Q.90. How will you treat Addison's disease?

Ans. Treatments are:

i. Glucocorticoid replacement:
Cortisol (hydrocortisone) is the drug of choice 15 mg in the morning and 5 mg at 6 PM.
Prednisolone—5 mg in morning and 2.5 mg in evening.

ii. Mineralocorticoid replacement:
Fludrocortisones (9 α-fluorohydrocortisone) is used. Usual dose is 0.05–0.1 mg daily.

Q.91. What advices would you give to patients on glucocorticoid replacement therapy?

Ans. Advices are:

i. Intercurrent stress—
   - Febrile illness: Double dose of hydrocortisone.

ii. Surgery—
   - Minor operation: Hydrocortisone 100 mg IM with premedication.
   - Major operation: Hydrocortisone 100 mg 6-hourly for 24 hours, then 50 mg IM 6-hourly until ready to take tablets.

iii. Vomiting—
   - Patients must have parenteral hydrocortisone if unable to take it by mouth.

iv. Steroid card—
   - Patient should carry this at all time. It should give information regarding diagnosis, steroid, dose, and doctor.

v. Bracelet—
   - Patients should be encouraged to buy one of these and have it engraved with the diagnosis and a reference number for a central database.

Q.92. What are the causes of polyuria and polydipsia?

Ans. Causes are:

- Diabetes mellitus
- Diabetes insipidus
- Hyperparathyroidism
- Conn's syndrome (hypokalemia).

Q.93. What is diabetes insipidus?

Ans. Diabetes insipidus is a disorder characterized by the persistent excretion of excessive quantities of dilute urine and by thirst.

Q.94. What are the types of diabetes insipidus?

Ans. Two types:

i. Cranial diabetes insipidus—It is due to deficient production of ADH by the hypothalamus.
ii. Nephrogenic diabetes insipidus—In which the renal tubules are unresponsive to ADH.

Q.95. How can you differentiate diabetes insipidus from diabetes mellitus?

Ans.

Character	Diabetes insipidus	Diabetes mellitus
Etiology	Deficiency of or unresponsive to ADH	Absolute or relative deficiency of insulin
Hyperglycemia	Absent	Present
Glycosuria	Absent	Present
Plasma osmolality	Low	Normal or high
Urine osmolality	Low	High
Urine sp. gravity	Low	High

Q.96. Mention some medical emergency in relation to endocrine disorder?

Ans. Medical emergencies are:

i. Hypoglycemia
ii. Diabetic ketoacidosis
iii. Pituitary apoplexy
iv. Thyrotoxic crisis
v. Addisonian crisis
vi. Severe hypercalcemia.

CHAPTER 9

Musculoskeletal Disease

Q.1. A 35-year-old lady presents with painful swelling of metacarpophalangeal, proximal interphalangeal joints of both hands and small joints of both feet for 3 months. What is your diagnosis?

Ans. Symmetrical polyarthritis is the diagnosis.

Q.2. What is polyarthritis?

Ans. Arthritis involving 5 or more joints is called polyarthritis.

Q.3. What is arthritis?

Ans. Arthritis means inflammation of joint. Joint is hot, swollen, and tender.

Q.4. What is arthralgia?

Ans. Arthralgia means painful joint. Joint is painful but not swollen and tender.

Q.5. What are the causes of polyarthritis?

Ans. Causes are:

- Rheumatoid arthritis
- Viral arthritis
- Systemic lupus erythematosus (SLE)
- Generalized osteoarthritis
- Seronegative spondyloarthritis (psoriasis, reactive, ankylosing spondylitis, enteropathic arthropathy)
- Chronic gout
- Juvenile idiopathic arthritis.

Q.6. What are the causes of symmetrical polyarthritis?

Ans. Causes are:

- Rheumatoid arthritis

- Viral arthritis
- Systemic lupus erythematosus (SLE)
- Generalized osteoarthritis
- Juvenile idiopathic arthritis.

Q.7. Which arthritides are more common in female?

Ans. All inflammatory arthritides are common in female except ankylosing spondylitis, reactive arthritis and gout which are more common in male.

Q.8. What is rheumatoid arthritis?

Ans. It is a chronic multisystem disorder of unknown etiology (autoimmune) characterized by bilateral symmetrical involvement of small peripheral joints and persisting inflammatory synovitis.

Q.9. What are the clinical patterns of presentation of rheumatoid arthritis?

Ans. Clinical patterns of presentation are:

i. Monocyclic: No further attack after 1st attack.
ii. Progressive: 20% of cases.
iii. Polycyclic: 70% of case with relapse and remissions.
iv. Palindromic: Monoarticular attacks lasting 24–48 hours.
v. Transient: Self-limiting lasting less than 12 hours.
vi. Chronic persistent: Most typical form. Once started does not end.
vii. Rapidly progressive: Rapidly progress over several years.

Q.10. Tell the diagnostic criteria for RA?

Ans. Criteria for the diagnosis of rheumatoid arthritis (American College of Rheumatology, 1987 revision)

- Morning stiffness > 1 hour
- Arthritis of three or more joints
- Arthritis of hand joints and wrists
- Symmetrical arthritis
- Subcutaneous nodules
- Positive serum rheumatoid factor
- Typical radiological changes (erosions and/or periarticular osteopenia).

First 1–4 for 6 weeks or more.

Four or more criteria are necessary for diagnosis.

Q.11. Please tell ACR-EULAR classification criteria.

Ans. In 2010, a collaborative effort between the American College of Rheumatology (ACR) and the European League Against Rheumatism (EULAR) revised the 1987 ACR classification criteria for RA in an effort to improve early diagnosis with the goal of identifying patients who would benefit from early introduction of disease modifying therapy.

Application of the newly revised criteria yields a score of 0–10, with a score of ≥6 fulfilling the requirements for definite RA.

Classification criteria for rheumatoid arthritis.

		Score
Joint involvement	1 large joint (shoulder, elbow, hip, knee, ankle)	0
	2–10 large joints	1
	1–3 small joints (MCP, PIP, thumb IP, MTP, wrists)	2
	4–10 small joints	3
	>10 joints (at least 1 small joint)	5
Serology	Negative RF and negative ACPA	0
	Low-positive RF or low-positive anti-CCP antibodies (3 times ULN)	2
	High-positive RF or high-positive anti-CCP antibodies (>3 times ULN)	3
Acute-phase reactants	Normal CRP and normal ESR	0
	Abnormal CRP or abnormal ESR	1
Duration of symptoms	<6 weeks	0
	6 weeks	1

Q.12. What are the common joint deformities develop in RA?

Ans. Hand joints—

i. Swan neck deformity (fixed flexion of the DIP and extension of PIP joints).
ii. Boutonniere/button hole deformity (fixed flexion of the PIP and extension of DIP joints).

iii. Z deformity of the thumb (hyperextension of the interphalangeal joint and fixed flexion and subluxation of metacarpophalangeal joint of the thumb).
iv. Triggering of fingers.
v. Ulnar deviation of hands.
vi. Dorsal subluxation of the ulna at the distal radioulnar joint.
vii. Radial deviation of wrist.

Foot joint—
Hammer toe deformity

Knee joint—
It may develop varus/valgus deformity.

Q.13. What are the ocular manifestations of RA?

Ans. Ocular manifestations are:
- Episcleritis
- Scleritis
- Scleromalacia
- Keratoconjunctivitis sicca (dryness of eyes and mouth).

Q.14. What are the cardiac manifestations of RA?

Ans. Cardiac manifestations are:
- Pericarditis
- Myocarditis
- Endocarditis
- Conduction defects
- Coronary vasculitis
- Granulomatous aortitis.

Q.15. What are the pulmonary manifestations of RA?

Ans. Pulmonary manifestations are:
- Nodules
- Pleural effusions
- Fibrosing alveolitis
- Bronchiolitis
- Caplan's syndrome.

Q.16. What are the neurological manifestations of RA?

Ans. Neurological manifestations are:
- Cervical cord compression
- Compression neuropathies (carpal tunnel syndrome)

- Peripheral neuropathy
- Mononeuritis multiplex.

Q.17. What is Caplan's syndrome?

Ans. Coal worker pneumoconiosis with rheumatoid nodules in the lung.

Q.18. What is Felty's syndrome?

Ans. Felty's syndrome is the association of splenomegaly and neutropenia with RA.

Q.19. Why does muscle wasting occur in RA?

Ans. Causes of muscle wasting are:

- Cytokines
- Prolonged disuse
- Nerve entrapment.

Q.20. What are the joints commonly involved in RA?

Ans. Almost all joints can be involved in RA except distal interphalangeal joints, lumbosacral spines.

Q.21. How many joint areas are included in ARA criteria?

Ans. 14 joint areas as below:

- Right and left upper limbs: PIP-2, MCP-2, wrist-2, elbow-2
- Right and left lower limbs: MTP-2, ankle-2, knee-2.

Q.22. What are the complications of RA?

Ans. Complications are:

i. Ruptured tendons
ii. Ruptured joints (Baker's cyst)
iii. Joint infection
iv. Spinal cord compression
v. Rarely amyloidosis
vi. Side effects of therapy
   - Dyspepsia
   - GI bleeding
   - Perforation
   - Anemia
   - Renal impairment
   - Bone marrow hypoplasia.

Q.23. What are differential diagnoses for early RA?

Ans. Differential diagnoses are:

- Postviral arthritis

- Systemic lupus erythematosus
- Seronegative spondarthritides
- Polymyalgia rheumatica
- Acute nodal osteoarthritis.

Q.24. What are the common viruses causing arthritis?

Ans. Rubella, hepatitis B or parvovirus are the common viruses causing arthritis.

Q.25. What investigations are done in RA?

Ans. Investigations are:

a. To establish diagnosis:
   i. ESR, CRP- raised.
   ii. Serology
      - RF positive in 70% cases
      - ANA at low titer in 30%
      - Anti CCP.
   iii. X-rays of affected joint
      - Soft tissue swelling
      - Periarticular osteopenia
      - Marginal nonproliferative erosions.
   iv. MRI
      - Demonstrations of early erosions.
   v. Aspirations of joint effusions.

b. To monitor drug safety:
   - CBC
   - Urinanalysis
   - LFT
   - Serum creatinine.

Q.26. What is rheumatoid factor?

Ans. Rheumatoid factor is an antibody directed against Fc portion of IgG. It may be IgM or IgG type. Rheumatoid factor is positive in 70% cases. We commonly measure IgM type but IgG type is more specific.

Q.27. What are the causes of anemia in RA?

Ans. Causes are:

i. Normocytic normochromic anemia (anemia of chronic disease, hemolytic anemia (Coomb's test may be positive), bone marrow suppression, splenomegaly).
ii. Microcytic hypochromic anemia (GI blood loss-NSAID).

iii. Macrocytic anemia (folate depletion—methotrexate therapy, associated with pernicious anemia).

Q.28. What are the radiological changes in RA?

Ans. Radiological changes are:

- Soft tissue swelling
- Periarticular osteopenia
- Marginal nonproliferative erosions
- Reduction of joint space
- Subluxation or bony ankylosis.

Q.29. What are the principles of management of RA?

Ans. Principles of management are:

- Relief of pain
- Reduction of inflammation
- Protection of articular structures
- Maintenance of function
- Control of systemic involvement.

Q.30. Tell the management of RA?

Ans. Management—

A. Nonpharmacological intervention
- Education
- Exercise
- Physical treatment
  - Physiotherapy
  - Hydrotherapy
  - Joint splinting.

B. Pharmacological therapy.

i. NSAIDs and analgesics to control symptoms.

ii. Glucocorticoids—Oral/intra-articular.

iii. DMARD-1st line—Methotrexate and sulfasalazine are used commonly.

iv. Cytokine neutralizing agents.

a. Anti TNF agents:
   - Infliximab
   - Etanercept
   - Adalimumab.

b. IL-I receptor antagonist:
   - Anakinra.

v. Immunosuppressive and cytotoxic drug.

C. Surgical

i. Synovectomy of wrist or finger tendon sheath (for pain relief/tendon rupture).
ii. In advanced or severe case—Osteotomy, arthrodesis, and anthroplasties.

Q.31. Tell a commonly used protocol for management of rheumatoid arthritis.

Ans. Commonly used protocol for management are:
- Establish the diagnosis clinically.
- Use NSAIDs and analgesics to control symptoms.
- Try to induce remission with IM depot methylprednisolone 80–120 mg if synovitis persists beyond 6 weeks.
- If synovitis recurs, refer to a rheumatologist to start sulfasalazine or methotrexate. Give a second dose of IM depot methylprednisolone.
- Refer for physiotherapy and general advice through a specialist team.
- If there is no significant improvement in 6–12 weeks as measured by less pain, less morning stiffness and reduced acute-phase response, use a combination of methotrexate and sulfasalazine.
- If no response, use an alternative agent, such as gold, d-penicillamine, leflunomide or Anti-TNF- α therapy.

Q.32. What is DMARD?

Ans. DMARD means disease-modifying antirheumatic drugs (DMARDs).

Q.33. When will you start DMARD?

Ans. As early as possible after diagnosis.

Q.34. How long DMARD should be continued?

Ans. There is no consensus that how long DMARD should be continued.

Q.35. What are the indications for DMARDs in the treatment of inflammatory rheumatic diseases?

Ans. The main indications for DMARDs are:
- Persistent inflammatory synovitis (> 6 weeks)
- Systemic vasculitis
- Systemic lupus erythematosus with cardiac, renal or CNS involvement
- As an adjunct to corticosteroid therapy in polymyalgia rheumatica and myositis.

Q.36. What are the most commonly used DMARD?

Ans. Methotrexate and sulfasalazine are the most commonly used DMARD.

Q.37. Please tell the name of some other DMARD.

Ans. Some other DMARD:

- Hydroxychloroquine
- Leflunomide
- Gold, penicillamine, and cyclosporine A.

Q.38. What are the side effects of methotrexate?

Ans. GI upset, stomatitis, rash, alopecia, hepatotoxicity, and acute pneumonitis are the side effects of methotrexate.

Q.39. Tell how methotrexate is prescribed in RA?

Ans. Initially 7.5 mg single dose weekly. The dose is gradually increased upto 25 mg weekly single dose. For prevention of side effect, folic acid is given the following day, e.g. methotrexate on Saturday, folic acid on Sunday.

Q.40. What are the side effects of sulfasalazine?

Ans. Nausea, GI upset, rash, hepatitis, neutropenia, and pancytopenia (rare) are the side effects of sulfasalazine.

Q.41. What are the indications of steroids in RA?

Ans. Principal indications for systemic corticosteroids are:

- Short-term control of inflammatory arthritis whilst awaiting efficacy from DMARD.
- Maintenance therapy in RA that cannot be adequately controlled by DMARD alone.
- Systemic vasculitis.
- Control of inflammatory disease during pregnancy.

Q.42. What are the indications of intra-articular steroid?

Ans. Monoarthritis—Better to avoid multiple joints and weight bearing joints, if a weight bearing joint causes more problems steroid is given.

Q.43. What are the newer drugs (biologic DMARD) used in treatment of RA?

Ans. Anti-TNF agents:

- Infliximab
- Etanercept
- Adalimumab

IL-I receptor antagonist:

- Anakinra
- Rituximab
- Abatacept
- Tocilizumab.

Q.44. What is the indication for giving newer biological agent for treatment of RA?

Ans. When there is no response to at least 2 conventional DMARD for optimum dose and duration, then a biological agent together with a DMARD is used.

Q.45. What are disadvantages of uses of biologic DMARD?

Ans.
i. They require subcutaneous or parenteral administration.
ii. Anti-TNF has the risk of serious infections, particularly reactivation of latent tuberculosis.
iii. There is also evidence of a possible increased risk of malignancy with use of anti-TNF.

Q.46. If RA untreated, then what will be the complications?

Ans. Joint destruction, deformity and disability will be the complications.

Q.47. How can you assess response to therapy?

Ans. i. Clinical— Reduction of joint swelling and pain
Morning stiffness less than or equal to 15 minutes
Reduction of joint tenderness.

ii. Laboratory—ESR↓
CRP↓.

Q.48. What are the poor prognostic factors for RA?

Ans. Poor prognostic factors are:

- Insidious onset
- Higher baseline disability
- Female gender
- Involvement of MTP joints
- Positive rheumatoid factor
- Blood very high ESR and CRP
- Disease duration over 3 months without treatment.

Q.49. What are the prognosis of RA?

Ans. Prognosis are:

- Lifespan reduced by 8–15 years
- 40% will be disabled within 3 years

- 80% will be disabled within 10 years
- If on treatment 20% complete remission.

Q.50. What are the connective tissue disorders?

Ans. Connective tissue disorders are:
- Systemic lupus erythematosus
- Systemic sclerosis
- Dermatomyositis
- Polymyositis.

Q.51. A 27-year-old lady presents with symmetrical arthritis of hand joints without any deformity for 6 months. She gives history of two spontaneous abortions. She has malar rash and oral ulcer. What is your diagnosis?

Ans. Systemic lupus erythematosus is the diagnosis.

Q.52. What are the types of arthritis in systemic lupus erythematosus?

Ans. Types of systemic lupus erythematosus are nonerosive and nondeforming symmetrical inflammatory polyarthritis.

Q.53. What are the diagnostic criteria for systemic lupus erythematosus?

Ans. Revised American Rheumatism Association criteria for systemic lupus erythematosus.

Features	Characteristics
Malar rash	Fixed erythema, flat or raised, sparing the nasolabial folds
Discoid rash	Erythematous raised patches with adherent keratotic scarring and follicular plugging
Photosensitivity	Rash due to unusual reaction to sunlight
Oral ulcers	Oral or nasopharyngeal ulceration, which may be painless
Arthritis	Nonerosive, involving two or more peripheral joints
Serositis	Pleuritis (history of pleuritic pain or rub, or pleural effusion) or pericarditis (rub, ECG evidence or effusion)
Renal disorder	Persistent proteinuria > 0.5 gm/day or cellular casts (red cell, granular or tubular)

Contd...

Contd...

Features	Characteristics
Neurological disorder	Seizures or psychosis, in the absence of provoking drugs or metabolic derangement
Hematological disorder	Hemolytic anemia or leukopenia (< 4 ×10^9/L), or lymphopenia (< 1 × 10^9/L), or thrombocytopenia (< 100 × 10^9/L) in the absence of offending drugs
Immunological disorder	Anti-DNA antibodies in abnormal titer or presence of antibody to Sm antigen or positive antiphospholipid antibodies
Antinuclear antibody (ANA) disorder	Abnormal titer of ANA by immunofluorescence

Q.54. How is the diagnosis of systemic lupus erythematosus made?

Ans. Presence of 4 or more criteria at a time or sequentially.

Q.55. What is anti-ds-DNA?

Ans. Anti ds-DNA means antibody to DNA (double-stranded). Anti-ds-DNA antibodies are characteristic of severe active SLE but occur in only around 30% of cases.

Q.56. What history would you take if you suspect systemic lupus erythematosus?

Ans. History of—

i. Whether the rash is aggravated on exposure to sunlight
ii. Raynaud's phenomenon
iii. Convulsion and psychiatric history
iv. Drugs and oral contraceptive pill
v. Family history of systemic lupus erythematosus
vi. Repeated abortion in female
vii. History of DVT and thromboembolism.

Q.57. What are the types of rash in systemic lupus erythematosus?

Ans. Three distinct types of rash occur:

i. The classic butterfly facial rash (upto 20% of patients).
ii. Subacute cutaneous lupus erythematosus (SCLE) rashes.
iii. Discoid lupus lesions.

Q.58. Describe a typical systemic lupus erythematosus rash.

Ans. This is an erythematous, raised and painful or itchy rash occurring over the cheeks with sparing of the nasolabial folds (the classic butterfly facial rash).

Q.59. What is Raynaud's phenomenon?

Ans. Raynaud's phenomenon is a syndrome of episodic digital ischemia manifested by triphasic color-pallor, cyanosis and redness of fingers and toes on exposure to cold.

Q.60. Please tell the goals of treatment of systemic lupus erythematosus.

Ans. Goals of treatment are:
- To educate the patient about the nature of the illness
- To control symptoms
- To prevent organ damage.

Q.61. What are the treatment for systemic lupus erythematosus?

Ans. a. General—
   i. Patients should be advised to avoid sun and UV light exposure, and to employ sun blocks.
   ii. Advise to stop smoking.
   iii. Control of cardiovascular risk factors, such as hypertension and hyperlipidemia.

b. Specific—
   i. Mild disease restricted to skin and joints—Analgesics and/or NSAIDs, and if necessary hydroxychloroquine (200–400 mg daily).
   ii. Moderate disease (such as rash, synovitis, pleurisy and pericarditis)—Short courses of oral steroids.
   iii. Life-threatening disease affecting the kidney, CNS or cardiovascular system—High-dose steroids and immunosuppressives. A commonly used regimen is pulse methylprednisolone (500 mg–1 gm IV) coupled with cyclophosphamide (2 mg/kg IV), repeated at 2–3 weekly intervals on 6–8 occasions, depending on the clinical response.

Q.62. What is the prognosis of systemic lupus erythematosus?

Ans. 5 years survival— 90%.

Q.63. What are the causes of death in systemic lupus erythematosus?

Ans. Causes are:

i. Renal failure
ii. Sepsis
iii. Premature cardiovascular disease.

Q.64. A 20-year-old man presents with painful swelling of both knee and right ankle joints for 2 weeks. What is your diagnosis?

Ans. Oligoarthritis is the diagnosis.

Q.65. What do you mean by oligoarthritis?

Ans. Arthritis involving 2–4 joints.

Q.66. What are the common causes of oligoarthritis?

Ans. Common causes are:

a. Seronegative spondyloarthritis
   i. Reactive arthritis
   ii. Psoriatic arthritis
   iii. Ankylosing spondylitis
   iv. Enteropathic arthritis.
b. Osteoarthritis
c. Juvenile idiopathic arthritis
d. Oligoarticular presentation of polyarthritis, e.g. RA.

Q.67. What are the types of seronegative spondyloarthritis?

Ans. Types are:

- Ankylosing spondylitis
- Reactive arthritis, including Reiter's syndrome
- Psoriatic arthritis
- Arthropathy associated with inflammatory bowel disease (enteropathic arthritis).

Q.68. What are the diagnostic criteria for seronegative spondyloarthritis?

Ans. i. Asymmetrical inflammatory oligoarthritis (lower > upper limb)
ii. Sacroiliitis and/or inflammatory spondylitis
iii. Inflammatory enthesitis
iv. Anterior uveitis
v. Tendency for familial aggregation (HLA B27)
vi. Persistently negative RF

vii. Absence of nodules and other extra-articular features of RA.

Q.69. What is ankylosing spondylitis?

Ans. Ankylosing spondylitis (AS) is characterized by a chronic inflammatory arthritis predominantly affecting the sacroiliac joints and spine, which can progress to bony fusion of the spine.

Q.70. What is the age and sex prevalence of AS?

Ans. Age and sex prevalence of AS are:
- Peak onset in the second or third decade
- Male: female ratio 3:1.

Q.71. What is genetic correlation of AS?

Ans. More than 90% of those affected are HLA-B27-positive.

Q.72. What is the most common presentation of AS?

Ans. Recurrent episodes of low back pain with marked morning and inactivity stiffness is the most common presentation of AS.

Q.73. What are the features of back pain in ankylosing spondylitis?

Ans. Features are:
- Morning stiffness >30 minutes.
- Improvement with exercise but not with rest.
- Awakening from back pain during only the second half of the night.
- Alternating buttock pain.

Q.74. What findings would you expect by examining the spine?

Ans. Findings are:
- Loss of lumbar lordosis, marked thoracic kyphosis, compensated cervical hyperextension.
- Tender over sacroiliac joints.
- Increased wall occiput distance.
- Restricted movement of spines in all direction.
- Positive Schober's test.

Q.75. What are the extra-articular features of ankylosing spondylitis?

Ans. Extra-articular features are:
- Plantar fasciitis

- Achilles tendenitis
- Anterior uveitis
- Aortic incompetence
- Cardiac conduction defects
- Pulmonary apical fibrosis.

Q.76. Does AS involve peripheral joints?

Ans. Yes.

Q.77. What is the pattern of peripheral arthritis?

Ans. Asymmetrical inflammatory oligoarthritis affecting hip, knee, ankles, and shoulders.

Q.78. What are the modified New York criteria (1984) for diagnosis for ankylosing spondylitis?

Ans. Modified New York criteria (1984) for diagnosis consist of the following:

1. History of inflammatory back pain
2. Limitation of motion of the lumbar spine in both the sagittal and frontal planes
3. Limited chest expansion
4. Definite radiographic sacroiliitis.

Criterion 4 plus any one of the other three criteria is sufficient for a diagnosis of definite AS.

Q.79. What are the radiological findings in sacroiliitis?

Ans. Sacroiliitis begins in the lower synovial parts of the joints with irregularity and loss of cortical margins leading to pseudowidening of the joint space and subsequently sclerosis, narrowing, and fusion.

Q.80. What are the radiological findings in lumbosacral spines?

Ans. Radiological findings are:

i. Straightening of lumbar spine caused by loss of lordosis.
ii. 'Squaring' of vertebrae due to erosion and sclerosis of the anterior corners of the vertebrae.
iii. Formation of bridging syndesmophytes.
iv. Ossification of the anterior longitudinal ligament and facet joint fusion.
v. The combination of all these features results in the typical 'bamboo' spine.

Q.81. Why is early diagnosis difficult in ankylosing spondylitis?

Ans. 1. Back pain is very common, but AS is much less common.

2. Diagnosis is clinical, little help from investigation. An early presumptive diagnosis often relies on clinical grounds requiring considerable expertise.
3. Young individuals with early AS are often reluctant to seek medical care.

Q.82. How can you differentiate ankylosing spondylitis from RA clinically?

Ans.

Ankylosing spondylitis	RA
Onset—2nd–3rd decade	More common in 4th–5th decade
More in male	More in female
Sacroiliitis, spondylitis, asymmetrical oligoarthritis involving large joints	Symmetrical polyarthritis involving small and large joints, no sacroiliitis or lower spine involvement
Uveitis	Scleritis

Q.83. How will you treat a case of ankylosing spondylitis?

Ans. Treatment:

i. Regular physical exercise. Swimming is ideal exercise. Poor posture must be avoided
ii. NSAIDs for relieving symptoms
iii. Sulfasalazine, methotrexate to control pheripheral arthritis
iv. Anti TNF therapy for disease inadequately controlled by above measures
v. Local corticosteroids—Plantar fasciitis
vi. Surgery—Severe hip, knee, ankle, shoulder restriction.

Q.84. An 18-year-old boy presents with painful swelling of left knee joint for 10 days. What is your diagnosis?

Ans. Monoarthritis of knee joint.

Q.85. What are the causes of monoarthritis?

Ans. i. Infective arthritis—Pyogenic
– Tuberculous

ii. Traumatic arthritis

iii. Monoarticular presentation of oligo-or polyarthritis
   - Reactive, psoriatic or other seronegative spondarthritis.
   - Rheumatoid arthritis.
   - Juvenile idiopathic arthritis.

iv. Hemarthrosis associated with clotting abnormality, e.g. hemophilia.

v. Crystal synovitis: Gout and pseudogout.

vi. Osteoarthritis.

Q.86. What may be the cause in this patient?

Ans. Causes are:
- Reactive arthritis
- Septic arthritis
- Tuberculous arthritis
- Traumatic arthritis.

Q.87. What history would you take if you suspect reactive arthritis?

Ans. History of bloody diarrhea, dysentery, and sexual exposure.

Q.88. What is reactive arthritis?

Ans. It is an inflammatory arthritis that typically affects young men following an episode of bloody diarrhea or sexual exposure.

Q.89. What are the organisms responsible for enteric acquired reactive arthritis?

Ans. Salmonella, Shigella, Campylobacter or Yersinia organisms are responsible for enteric acquired reactive arthritis.

Q.90. What is the organism responsible for sexually acquired reactive arthritis?

Ans. Chlamydia is the organism responsible for sexually aquired reactive arthritis.

Q.91. Please tell the clinical features of reactive arthritis.

Ans. Clinical features are:

i. Acute onset inflammatory oligoarthritis affecting large joints of lower limbs 1–3 weeks following sexual exposure or an attack of dysentery.

ii. Additional extra-articular features:
   - Circinate balanitis

- Keratoderma blennorrhagica
- Nail dystrophy
- Oral ulcer
- Uveitis.

Q.92. What is Reiter's syndrome?

Ans. It is a triad of

- Nonspecific urethritis
- Conjunctivitis
- Reactive arthritis.

Q.93. How can you treat reactive arthritis?

Ans. Treatment—

i. Rest.
ii. NSAIDs and analgesics for relieve of pain.
iii. Intra-articular injection of corticosteroids for marked synovitis.
iv. DMARDs for patients with persistent marked symptoms, recurrent arthritis or severe keratoderma blennorrhagica.
v. Anterior uveitis is treated as a medical emergency with topical, subconjunctival or systemic corticosteroids.

Q.94. What are the organisms responsible for septic arthritis?

Ans. In adults—*Staphylococcus aureus.*

In the elderly and intravenous drug misusers—Gram-negative bacilli or group B, C and G streptococci.

Q.95. How will you treat septic arthritis?

Ans. i. Admission of patient to hospital.
ii. Urgent investigations should be done.
iii. Intravenous antibiotic—Flucloxacillin 2 gm 6-hourly
   - If penicillin-allergic, give clindamycin 450–600 mg 6-hourly.
   - If at high risk of gram-negative sepsis (e.g. elderly, frail, recurrent urinary tract infection), add a cephalosporin (e.g. cefuroxime 1.5 gm 8-hourly).
iv. Relieve of pain—Oral and/or intravenous analgesics
   - Consider local ice-packs.
v. Decompression of joint—Serial needle aspiration to dryness (1–3 times/day as required).
vi. Physiotherapy from first day—Early regular passive movement, progressing to active movements once pain controlled and effusion not reaccumulating.

Q.96. A 34-year-old male presents with arthritis of DIP joints of both hands with erythematous scaly lesions in elbow and knees. What is the diagnosis?

Ans. Psoriatic arthritis is the diagnosis.

Q.97. What are the arthritis involving DIP joints?

Ans. Gout, osteoarthritis, and psoriasis are the arthritis involving DIP joints.

Q.98. What are the types of psoriatic arthritis?

Ans. Types are:
- Asymmetrical inflammatory oligoarthritis (40%)
- Symmetrical polyarthritis (25%)
- Distal IPJ arthritis
- Psoriatic spondylitis
- Arthritis mutilans.

Q.99. What are the nail changes in psoriasis?

Ans. Nail changes include pitting, onycholysis, subungual hyperkeratosis and horizontal ridging.

Q.100. What are the causes of arthritis mutilans?

Ans. Types are:
- Psoriatic arthritis
- Rheumatoid arthritis.

Q.101. A 60-year-old male presents with pain in both knees causing difficulty in sitting toilet and pain worsen in activity, lessened by rest. What is your diagnosis?

Ans. Osteoarthritis is the diagnosis.

Q.102. How can you differentiate mechanical arthritis from inflammatory arthritis?

Ans.

Features	Mechanical arthritis	Inflammatory arthritis
Age	Any age	Below 40 years
Onset	Acute	Insidious
Family history	Absent	Usually positive
Morning stiffness	Absent	Present
Rest	Better	Worse

Contd...

Contd...

Features	Mechanical arthritis	Inflammatory arthritis
Activity	Worse	Improved
Signs of inflammation	Absent	Present

Q.103. What are the causes of low back pain?

Ans. Causes are:
- Mechanical back pain (>90%).
- Nonmechanical back pain, e.g. malignancy, fracture, and infection.
- Inflammatory, e.g. seronegative spondyloarthritis.
- Other specific causes, e.g. prolapsed intervertebral disk prolapse.

Q.104. What are the features of simple mechanical low back pain?

Ans. Features are:
- Pain varies with physical activity (improved with rest)
- Sudden onset, precipitated by lifting or bending
- Recurrent episodes
- Pain limited to back or upper leg
- No clear-cut nerve root distribution
- No systemic features
- Prognosis good (90% recovery at 6 weeks).

Q.105. What are the specific causes of low back pain?

Ans. Specific causes are:
- Spondylolysis
- Spondylolisthesis
- Spinal stenosis
- Prolapsed intervertebral disk
- Arachnoiditis
- Vertebral fracture.

Q.106. Define osteoporosis.

Ans. Osteoporosis is defined as reduced bone density, which causes a micro-architectural deterioration of bone tissue and leads to an increased risk of fracture.

Q.107. Please tell the WHO classification of osteoporosis.

Ans. BMD

T-score >–1.0	Normal
–1.0 – –2.5	Osteopenia
<–2.5	Osteoporosis.

Q.108. Who are more prone to develop osteoporosis?

Ans. Postmenopausal women are more prone to develop osteoporosis.

Q.109. What is commonly used drug in the treatment of osteoporosis?

Ans. Bisphosphonate is the commonly used drug in the treatment of osteoporosis.

CHAPTER 10

Nervous System

Q.1. What do you mean by lower motor neuron?

Ans. Anterior horn cells of the spinal cord and cranial motor nerve nuclei in the brainstem with their axons are known as lower motor neuron.

Q.2. What do you mean by upper motor neuron?

Ans. The pyramidal cells of the cerebral cortex (motor area) with its axons are known as upper motor neuron.

Q.3. What are the differences between UMN and LMN lesion?

Ans.

Clinical signs	Upper motor lesion	Lower motor lesion
Power	Weak Upper limbs: extensors weaker Lower limbs: flexors weaker	Weak
Wasting	None	Yes
Fasciculation	None	Yes
Tone	Spastic increase	Flaccid from onset
Reflexes	Increased	Reduced/ absent
Plantar response	Extensor	Flexor

Q.4. What is reflex?

Ans. Involuntary motor response in response to sensory stimulus.

Q.5. What are the types of reflex?

Ans. Types are:

- Superficial reflex
- Deep reflex.

Q.6. What are the root values of tendon reflexes?

Ans.

Reflex	Root value
A. Upper limb	
i. Biceps jerk	C_5/C_6
ii. Supinator jerk	C_5/C_6
iii. Triceps jerk	C_7
iv. Finger jerk	C_8
B. Lower limb	
i. Knee jerk	L_3/L_4
ii. Ankle jerk	S_1/S_2

Q.7. What are the causes of extensor plantar response?

Ans. Causes are:

i. Physiological
  - 1st year of life
  - Sleep

ii. Pathological
  - UMN lesion
  - Deep coma
  - Postictal period.

Q.8. What are the causes of absent ankle jerk but extensor plantar response?

Ans. Causes are:

- Subacute combined degeneration of spinal cord
- Multiple sclerosis
- Friedreich's ataxia
- Diabetes mellitus with cervical spondylosis.

Q.9. What are the features of 3rd nerve palsy?

Ans. Features are:

- Complete ptosis
- Eyeball deviated to outward (divergent squint)
- Dilated pupil nonreacting to light and unable to move upward, downward, and medially.

Q.10. What is the common symptom of 3rd nerve palsy?

Ans. Diplopia is the common symptom of 3rd nerve palsy.

Q.11. What are the causes of ptosis?

Ans. Causes are:

- 3rd nerve palsy
- Horner's syndrome
- Myasthenia gravis
- Myopathy
- Mechanical ptosis, e.g. eyelid tumor.

Q.12. What are the features of Horner's syndrome?

Ans. Features are:

- Partial ptosis
- Meiosis (small pupil)
- Anhidrosis (ipsilateral failure of sweating)
- Enophthalmos.

Q.13. What are the causes of Horner's syndrome?

Ans. Causes are:

- Central (hypothalamus/brainstem)
- Peripheral (lung apex, carotid artery pathology)
- Idiopathic.

Q.14. What is Bell's palsy?

Ans. It is an idiopathic lower motor neuron type of facial nerve palsy. It may be related to viral infection, due to reactivation of latent herpes simplex virus 1.

Q.15. Where is the site of lesion in Bell's palsy?

Ans. Facial canal in the petrous part of temporal bone (just above stylomastoid foramen).

Q.16. What are the common presentations of Bell's palsy?

Ans. Common presentations are:

i. Usually in the morning, bystander notice asymmetry of face—Loss of nasolabial fold, deviation of angle of mouth towards healthy side.
ii. Patient complaints, dribbling of saliva and water from the angle of the mouth on the affected side.
iii. Accumulation of food particles between the gum and cheek.

Q.17. What are the findings on examination in Bell's palsy?

Ans. Findings are:

- Facial asymmetry.
- Loss of the nasolabial fold.

- Absence of wrinkling of forehead.
- Unable to close the eye.
- Bell's phenomenon present.
- Unable to puff the cheek, failure to wistle and smile.
- Deviation of angle of mouth toward the healthy side on attempting to show teeth.
- Loss of taste sensation on the anterior 2/3rd of the tongue on the affected side.
- Hyperacusis may be present if lesion occurs within the facial canal.

Q.18. What is Bell's phenomenon?

Ans. On attempting to close the eyes, the eyeball is rolled upward and outward. This is called Bell's phenomenon.

Q.19. What is the difference between Bell's palsy and lower motor neuron facial palsy?

Ans. Bell's phenomenon is present in Bell's palsy but absent in LMN facial palsy.

Q.20. How will you treat a case of Bell's palsy?

Ans. Treatments:

i. Prednisolone 40–60 mg daily plus acyclovir for 1 week should be given within 72 hours.
ii. Artificial tears and ointment prevent exposure keratitis and the eye should be taped shut overnight.
iii. Physiotherapy—Facial exercise, electrostimulation within 14 days.

Q.21. How can you differentiate UMN and LMN facial palsy?

Ans.

UMN VIIth nerve palsy	LMN VIIth nerve palsy
Contralateral lower-half of face is involved	Ipsilateral half (both lower and upper) of face is involved
Wrinkling of forehead and closing of eye are spared	Wrinkling of forehead and closing of eye are involved

Q.22. What is the most common cause of UMN facial palsy?

Ans. CVD is the most common cause of UMN facial palsy.

Q.23. What is bulbar palsy?

Ans. Bulbar palsy is the lower motor neuron lesion of X, XI, XIIth cranial nerves.

Q.24. What are the causes of bulbar palsy?

Ans. Causes are:

- Poliomyelitis
- Motor neurone disease
- Syringobulbia
- Medullary infarction
- Brainstem tumors
- Myasthenia
- Guillain-Barré syndrome.

Q.25. What is pseudobulbar palsy?

Ans. Pseudobulbar palsy is UMN lesion of X, XI, XIIth cranial nerves resulting from bilateral lesion of corticobulbar pathways.

Q.26. What are the causes of pseudobulbar palsy?

Ans. Causes are:

- Bilateral hemisphere (lacunar) infarction
- Motor neuron disease
- Multiple sclerosis
- High brainstem tumors.

Q.27. How can you differentiate bulbar and pseudobulbar palsy?

Ans.

Pseudobulbar palsy	Bulbar palsy
Lesion of corticobulbar pathways to V,VII,X,XI,XII	Lesion to X, XI, XII
Bilateral UMN	LMN lesion
Small spastic tongue	Wasted fasciculating tongue
Jaw jerk exaggerated	Jaw jerk normal
Spastic dysarthria	Nasal speech and regurgitation

Q.28. What is headache?

Ans. Headache is the pain in and around the vertex.

Q.29. What are the common headaches?

Ans. Common headaches are:

- Tension headache
- Migraine
- Cluster headache

- Referred headache
- Headache of raised intracranial pressure.

Q.30. Describe a tension type headache.

Ans. Tension type headache is described as 'dull', 'tight' or like a 'pressure', or a sensation of a band round the head or pressure at the vertex.

Q.31. Describe an attack of classical migraine.

Ans. A classical migraine attack starts with a nonspecific prodrome of malaise and irritability followed by the aura of a focal neurological event (usually visual), and then a severe, throbbing, hemicranial headache with photophobia and vomiting.

Q.32. How can you treat a migraine attack?

Ans. Simple analgesia with aspirin or paracetamol, combined with an antiemetic such as metoclopramide or domperidone.

Q.33. What are the drugs used to prevent recurrent attacks of migraine?

Ans. Drugs are:

- Pizotifen
- Propranolol
- Amitriptyline
- Sodium valproate
- Topiramate.

Q.34. Describe an attack of cluster headache.

Ans. Periodic, severe, unilateral periorbital pain accompanied by unilateral lacrimation, nasal congestion and conjunctival injection lasting for 30–90 minutes at a particular time of the day for several days after interval of weeks to months.

Q.35. What are the characteristics of headache of raised intracranial pressure?

Ans. Characteristics are:

- Worse in morning, improves through the day
- Associated with morning vomiting
- Worse bending forward
- Worse with cough and straining
- Relieved by analgesia
- Dull ache, often mild.

Q.36. Define seizure.

Ans. Seizure is a paroxysmal event due to abnormal, excessive, hypersynchronous discharges from an aggregate of CNS neurons.

Q.37. Define epilepsy.

Ans. Epilepsy may be defined as a tendency to have recurrent seizures.

Q.38. Define convulsion.

Ans. Motor component of a seizure is known as convulsion.

Q.39. What are the types of epilepsy according to seizure type?

Ans. Types of epilepsy according to seizure type:

i. Partial (simple or complex)
ii. Partial with secondary generalization
iii. Primary generalized
   - Tonic-clonic
   - Absence
   - Tonic
   - Atonic
   - Myoclonic.

Q.40. What are the stages of tonic-clonic seizure?

Ans. Stages are:

i. Prodormal phase: It may be irritable for some days before seizure.
ii. Aura: A tonic-clonic seizure may be preceded by a partial seizure—The 'aura'.
iii. Tonic phase: The patient then goes rigid and becomes unconscious, falling down heavily if standing and often sustaining an injury. During this phase, respiration is arrested and central cyanosis may be witnessed.
iv. Clonic phase: After a few moments, the rigidity is periodically relaxed, producing clonic jerks. During the attack, urinary incontinence may occur, as may tounge biting. A severly bitten, bleeding tongue after an attack of loss of consciousness is pathognomonic of a generalized seizure.
v. Postictal phase: The patient then gradually regains consciousness, but is in a confused and disoriented

state for half an hour or more after regaining consciousness. Full memory function may not be recovered for some hours. After a generalized seizure the patient usually feels terrible, may have a headache and will want to sleep.

Q.41. What are the Trigger factors for seizures?

Ans. Trigger factors are:

- Sleep deprivation
- Alcohol (particularly withdrawal)
- Recreational drug misuse
- Physical and mental exhaustion
- Flickering lights, including TV and computer screens (primary generalized epilepsies only)
- Intercurrent infections and metabolic disturbances
- Uncommonly: Loud noises, music, reading, and hot baths.

Q.42. How can you differentiate seizure from syncope?

Ans.

Point	Seizure	Syncope
Aura(e.g. olfactory)	Present	Absent
Cyanosis	Present	Absent
Tongue biting	Present	Absent
Postictal confusion	Present	Absent
Postictal amnesia	Present	Absent
Postictal headache	Present	Absent
Rapid recovery	No	Yes

Q.43. How can you differentiate epileptic fit and hysterical fit?

Ans.

Traits	Hysterical convulsion	Epileptic convulsion
Age	Young age	Any age
Sex	More in females	Both sexes are equally affected

Contd...

Contd...

Traits	Hysterical convulsion	Epileptic convulsion
Consciousness	No real loss of consciousness.	Real loss of consciousness
Convulsion	Pseudoconvulsion	True convulsion
Time and place of fit	In presence of family member and never during sleep	At any time and any place
Duration	Persists for long duration	Short duration
Tongue bite and urinary incontinence	Absent	Present
Eyeball	Rolling	Fixed
Postictal confusion, headache, amnesia	Absent	Present

Q.44. How to administer first aid measures for seizures.

Ans.
- i. Move person away from danger (fire, water, machinery, and furniture).
- ii. After convulsions cease, turn into 'recovery' position (semi-prone).
- iii. Ensure airway is clear, but do not insert anything in mouth (tongue biting occurs at seizure onset and cannot be prevented by observers).
- iv. If convulsions continue for more than 5 minutes or recur without person regaining consciousness, summon urgent medical attention.
- v. Do not leave person alone until fully recovered (drowsiness and confusion can persist for upto 1 hour).

Q.45. Please tell immediate management of seizures.

Ans. Immediate management of seizures—
- i. Ensure airway is patent.
- ii. Give oxygen to offset cerebral hypoxia.

iii. Give intravenous anticonvulsant (e.g. diazepam 10 mg) only if convulsions are continuous or repeated (if so, manage as for status epilepticus).
iv. Take blood for anticonvulsant levels (if known epileptic).
v. Investigate cause.

Q.46. Please tell the initial management of status epilepticus.

Ans. Initial management of status epilepticus—

i. Ensure airway is patent, give oxygen to prevent cerebral hypoxia, and secure intravenous access.
ii. Draw blood for glucose, urea, and electrolytes (including Ca and Mg), and liver function, and store a sample for future analysis (e.g. drug misuse).
iii. Give diazepam 10 mg IV (or rectally) or lorazepam 4 mg IV—Repeat once only after 15 minutes.
iv. Transfer to intensive care area, monitoring neurological condition, blood pressure, respiration and blood gases, intubating and ventilating patient if appropriate.

Q.47. What is the first line drug for partial and/or secondary GTCS?

Ans. Carbamazepine is the first line drugs for partial and/or secondary GTCS.

Q.48. What is the first line drug for absence seizure?

Ans. Ethosuximide is the first line drug for absence seizure.

Q.49. What is the first line drug for primary GTCS?

Ans. Sodium valproate is the first line drug for primary GTCS.

Q.50. What is acute confusional state (delirium)?

Ans. Acute confusional state (delirium) is defined as a global impairment of cognitive function with disturbance of arousal.

Q.51. What are the common causes of acute confusional state?

Ans. Common causes of acute confusional state are—

i. Infective
   - Chest infection
   - Urinary infection
   - Septicemia
   - Viral illness

- Meningitis
- Encephalitis.

ii. Metabolic/endocrine
- Hypoxia (respiratory failure)
- Hyper-/hypoglycemia
- Hyponatremia
- Liver failure and renal failure.

iii. Vascular
- Acute cerebral hemorrhage/infarction
- Subarachnoid hemorrhage.

iv. Toxic
- Alcohol intoxication/withdrawal
- Drugs (therapeutic/illicit).

iv. Neoplastic
- Secondary deposits.

v. Trauma
- Head injury (cerebral contusions)
- Subdural hematoma.

Q.52. What is dementia?

Ans. It is defined as a global impairment of cognitive function without alteration of consciousness and memory is most affected in the early stages.

Q.53. What are the causes of dementia?

Ans. Causes of dementia are:

i. Vascular
- Diffuse small vessel disease.

ii. Degenerative/inherited
- Alzheimer's disease
- Huntington's disease
- Wilson's disease
- Pick's disease
- Cortical Lewy body disease.

iii. Neoplastic
- Secondary deposits
- Primary cerebral tumor.

iv. Traumatic
- Chronic subdural hematoma.

v. Toxic/nutritional
- Alcohol
- Thiamine deficiency

- B_{12} deficiency
- Hypothyroidism.

Q.54. What are the reversible causes of dementia?

Ans. Reversible causes of dementia are remembered by the mnemonics DEMENTIA:

D—Drugs (any drug with anticholinergic activity)
E— Emotional (depression)
M— Metabolic (hypoxia)
E— Endocrine(hypothyroid)
N—Normal pressure hydrocephalus
T— Tumor or other space-occupying lesion
I— Infection (syphilis, AIDS)
A— Anemia (vitamin B_{12} or folate deficiency), vitamin B_1 deficiency also.

Q.55. What is coma?

Ans. Coma is defined as persistent loss of consciousness.

Q.56. What are the causes of unconsciousness (coma)?

Ans. Common causes of coma (remember by mnemonics—AEIOU, DAMM)

AEIOU

A—Alcohol and abscess
E— Epilepsy, encephalitis, endocrine, and electrolyte disturbance
I—Head injury and brainstem infarction or hemorrhage
O—Opium and drug overdose
U— Uremia.

DAMM

D—Diabetes (hypoglycemia, diabetic ketoacidosis, non-ketotic hyperosmolar hyperglycemia)
A—Apoplexy, epidural and subdural hemorrhage, and subarachnoid hemorrhage
M—Meningitis and cerebral malaria
M—Metabolic (hepatic failure).

Q.57. What is stroke?

Ans. WHO definition of stroke: Stroke may be defined as a sudden onset of focal or global neurological deficit, which is nontraumatic vascular in origin, lasting more than 24 hours or die within this period and death cannot be attributed by any other events or imaging study done within 24 hours reveals infarction or hemorrhage.

Q.58. Classify stroke

Ans. Classifications:

1. On the basis of duration and evolution of symptoms—
   a. Transient ischemic attack
   b. Progressing stroke (stroke in evolution)
   c. Completed stroke.
2. Pathological classifications
   a. Infarctive/ ischemic stroke
   b. Hemorrhagic stroke
      - Primary intracerebral hemorrrhage
      - Subarachnoid hemorrhage (SAH).

Q.59. What is TIA?

Ans. Transient ischemic attack is a sudden onset of focal neurological deficit lasting minute to hours usually less than 24 hours with complete recovery.

Q.60. What are the major risk factors of stroke?

Ans. Major risk factors are:

- Smoking
- Hypertension
- Diabetes mellitus
- Hyperlipidemia
- Heart disease (atrial fibrillation, heart failure, and endocarditis).

Q.61. What are the common presentations of the stroke?

Ans. Depends on which artery is involved and which segment is involved—

i. Impaired consciousness/coma
ii. Hemiparesis or hemiplegia
iii. Hemisensory loss
iv. Aphasia
v. Visual field defect
vi. Brainstem deficit.

Q.62. What do you mean by paresis, plegia, hemiplegia, and paraplegia?

Ans. Paresis—Partial paralysis
Plegia—Complete paralysis
Hemiplegia—Paralysis of one-half of the body
Paraplegia—Paralysis of lower limbs.

Q.63. What is the common presentation of SAH?

Ans. Subarachnoid hemorrhage typically presents with a sudden, severe 'thunderclap' headache (often occipital) which lasts for hours or even days, often accompanied by vomiting.

Q.64. How will you differentiate between hemorrhagic and ischemic stroke clinically?

Ans. It is very difficult to differentiate clinically but the combination of severe headache and vomiting at the onset of the focal neurological deficits increases the likelihood of a hemorrhagic stroke.

Q.65. What are the investigations done in case of stroke?

Ans. Imaging: Brain CT scan (to see cerebrum) and MRI (to see cerebellum, brainstem).

If any hemorrhage is suspected, do it after 2–3 hours.
If infarction suspected, do it after 24 hours.

- ECG
- Blood glucose
- Lipid profile
- Blood for Hb%
- Urine R/M/E
- Serum creatinine
- Others, according to suspicion.

Q.66. Please tell the general measures of a stroke patient.

Ans. General management

i. Immediate hospitalization
ii. ABC management
   a. Airway: Keep patient in recovery position, clear airway.
   b. Breathing: Use oxygen or artificial respiration if required. Indicated if ($SaO_2 < 93\%$, hypotensive, etc.).
   c. Circulation maintenance.
iii. Nutrition—NPO initially; give feeding with NG tube every 2 hourly until swallowing assessed.
iv. General care
   a. Care of the bowel: Bowel movement at least once in a day.
   b. Care of the bladder: For unconscious patient with condom or indwelling catheter.

c. Care of eye and nose: Chloramphenicol eyedrop to prevent exposure keratitis.
d. Care of mouth: Use antifungal to prevent oral thrush.
e. Care of paralyzed part of the body: 2 hourly change of posture and regular physiotherapy to prevent bedsore or contracture.

Q.67. What are the specific measures for infarctive stroke?

Ans. For reperfusion of ischemic area—

i. Antiplatelet drugs—Aspirin, clopidogrel
ii. Intra-arterial thrombolysis
Use of r-tpA
iii. Modification of risk factors
iv. Treatment of complication.

Q.68. What are the complications of stroke?

Ans. Complications are:

- Chest infection
- Epileptic seizures
- Deep vein thrombosis / pulmonary embolism
- Frozen shoulder
- Pressure sores
- Urinary infection
- Constipation
- Depression and anxiety.

Q.69. What are the specific measures for hemorrhagic stroke?

Ans. Hemorrhagic stroke:

i. Hypertension should be controlled.
ii. Nimodipine is given to prevent vasospasm if ventricular extension is present.
iii. Anticoagulant or antiplatelet drugs are contraindicated.
iv. Surgical clot evacuation when—
a. Supratentorial hemorrhage: Hematoma >5 cm or hematoma 3–5 cm but deterioration of consciousness.
b. Infratentorial hemorrhage: Hematoma >5 cm or blood in ventricle.

Q.70. How can you treat TIA?

Ans. Treatments of TIA:

i. Antiplatelet—Aspirin
ii. Control of risk factors
iii. For carotid TIA, carotid Doppler study—If significant stenosis (>70% stenosis), carotid angiogram, and endarterectomy.

Q.71. What is Weber's syndrome?

Ans. Weber syndrome is a brainstem syndrome due to lesion in anterior cerebral peduncle (midbrain) characterized by—(a) Ipsilateral 3rd palsy, (b) contralateral upper motor neuron 7th palsy, and (c) contralateral hemiplegia.

Q.72. What is Millard-Gubler syndrome?

Ans. Millard-Gubler syndrome is a brainstem syndrome due to lesion in pontomedullary junction characterized by—(a) Ipsilateral 6th palsy, (b) ipsilateral lower motor neuron 7th palsy, and (c) contralateral hemiplegia.

Q.73. What is the investigation protocol for suspected subarachnoid hemorrhage?

Ans. Emergency CT→ i. Presence of blood in subarachnoid space and cisterns—SAH

↓

Negative→Lumbar puncture after 12 hours→ Xanthochromia / Blood— SAH

NB. If CT and CSF at 12 hours are negative, no SAH.

Q.74. How can you treat SAH?

Ans. Treatments of SAH:
- Referral to neurosurgeon
- Resuscitation
- Nimodipine 60 mg.

Q.75. A 22-year-old male patient presented with sudden onset of spastic paraparesis with definite sensory level and urinary retention. What are your diagnoses?

Ans. Diagnoses are:
- Spinal cord compression
- Acute transverse myelitis.

Q.76. What are the treatments of acute transverse myelitis?

Ans. Treatments are:
- High-dose intravenous methyl prednisolone.
- Supportive measure for a paralyzed patient.

Q.77. What are the causes of spinal cord compression?

Ans. Causes are:
- Trauma
- Tumors, e.g. meningioma, metastatic carcinoma (e.g. breast, prostate, bronchus), and myeloma
- Tuberculosis.

Q.78. What are the causes of spastic paraplegia?

Ans. Causes are:
- Spinal cord compression
- Acute transverse myelitis
- Multiple sclerosis
- Motor neuron disease
- Friedreich's ataxia
- Hereditary spastic paraplegia.

Q.79. What is the common chronic infection causing paraplegia?

Ans. Spinal tuberculosis (Pott's disease) is the common chronic infection causing paraplegia.

Q.80. A 15-year-old boy presented with weakness of both lower limb for 3 days which is ascending in nature. He has history of loose watery motion 14 days back. What is your most probable diagnosis?

Ans. Guillain-Barré syndrome is the most probable diagnosis.

Q.81. Which type of disease is Guillain-Barré syndrome?

Ans. Guillain-Barré syndrome is a immune-mediated acute inflammatory demyelinating polyneuropathy type of disease.

Q.82. Which type of paralysis occurs in Guillain-Barré syndrome?

Ans. Flaccid paralysis occurs in Guillain-Barré syndrome.

Q.83. What are the differential diagnoses of flaccid paralysis?

Ans. Differential diagnoses are:
- Guillain-Barré syndrome
- Poliomyelitis
- Botulism
- Hypo/hyperkalemic periodic paralysis.

Q.84. How can you differentiate GBS from poliomyelitis?

Ans. In GBS symmetrical involvement and in poliomyelitis asymmetrical involvement.

Q.85. What is the finding in poliomyelitis?

Ans. Asymmetric flaccid paralysis is the finding in poliomyelitis.

Q.86. What are the cardinal findings on examination of GBS patient?

Ans. Diffuse weakness with widespread loss of jerks.

Q.87. What is the condition of jerks in GBS?

Ans. Diminished or absent jerks.

Q.88. What are the investigations done in GBS?

Ans. Investigations are:

i. Lumbar puncture and CSF study
ii. Electrophysiological studies
iii. Investigation to identify an underlying cause, such as cytomegalovirus, mycoplasma or campylobacter, requires a chest X-ray, stool culture, and appropriate immunological blood tests.

Q.89. When will you do lumbar puncture?

Ans. 10 days after onset of disease.

Q.90. What are the typical findings in CSF?

Ans. Albuminocytological disassociation.

Q.91. What do you mean by albuminocytological disassociation?

Ans. CSF protein is elevated but usually no or little rise in CSF cell number.

Q.92. Please tell treatment of GBS.

Ans. Treatments are:

i. Hospitalization—Ideally the patient should be treated in ICU, may require artificial ventilation.
ii. High dose IV immunoglobulin (400 mg/kg/day for 5 days)—Shorten the duration of ventilation and improve prognosis, provided treatment is started within 14 days of the onset of symptoms.
iii. Plasmapheresis is equally effective.
iv. Physiotherapy is the mainstay of therapy after initial phase.

NB. Steroid is ineffective.

Q.93. What are the prognoses?

Ans. Prognoses are:

- 80% complete recovery

- 16% live with residual disability
- 4% die.

Q.94. What are the causes of sudden muscle weakness?

Ans. Causes are:

- GBS
- Poliomyelitis
- Botulism
- Stroke
- Hypo/hyperkalemic periodic paralysis.

Q.95. What are the common causes of peripheral neuropathy?

Ans. Common causes are:

(Remember ABCDI)

i. Alcohol
ii. Vit B_1, B_6 and B_{12} deficiency
iii. Carcinoma, chronic renal failure
iv. DM
v. Drugs— Isoniazid
   Ethambutol
   Metronidazole.
vi. Infections — Leprosy, HIV, and diphtheria.

Q.96. What are the common presentations of peripheral polyneuropathy?

Ans. Numbness, pain, and paresthesia in globe and stocking distribution, and distal weakness are the common presentations of peripheral polyneuropathy.

Q.97. What are your expected findings on examination?

Ans. Wasting, reduced muscle power, diminished or absent reflexes, and diminished all modalities of sensation are the expected findings on examinations.

Q.98. What are the causes of loss of tendon reflexes?

Ans. Causes are:

- Lower motor neuron lesion
- Peripheral neuropathy
- Dorsal column lesion
- Neuronal shock
- Hypo or hyperkalemia.

Q.99. How can you differentiate between neuropathy and myopathy?

Ans.

Trait	Neuropathy	Myopathy
Sensory symptom	May be present	Absent
Pattern of weakness	Predominately distal	Predominately proximal
Wasting	May be severe	Absent until late stage
Tone	Decreased/Increased	Normal usually
Involuntary movement	Present	Absent
Plantar	May be extensor	Flexor
Co-ordination	May be lost	Intact
Sensory function	Impaired	Intact

Q.100. Please name some drugs used to treat neuropathic pain.

Ans. Gabapentine, pregabalin, carbamazepine, and amitriptyline are some drugs used to treat neuropathic pain.

Q.101. An 18-year-old boy presented with high grade fever and headache for 3 days. On examination the boy is conscious, toxic and has stiff neck. What is your diagnosis?

Ans. Diagnosis is meningitis.

Q.102. What is meningitis?

Ans. Meningitis means inflammation of meninges. It is usually due to acute infection of the meninges which presents with a characteristic combination of pyrexia, headache, and meningism.

Q.103. What do you mean by meningism?

Ans. It consists of headache, photophobia, and signs of meningeal irritation:

i. Neck rigidity.

ii. Kernig's sign: It is the extension at the knee with the hip joint flexed causes spasm in the hamstring muscles.

iii. Brudzinski's sign: Passive flexion of the neck causes flexion of the hips and knees.

Q.104. What are the causes of neck stiffness?

Ans. Causes are:

i. Meningitis
ii. Subarachnoid hemorrhage
iii. Cervical spondylitis
iv. Tetanus.

Q.105. What are the common causes of meningitis?

Ans. Common causes are:

- Viral meningitis
- Bacterial meningitis
- Tuberculous meningitis.

Q.106. Please tell the parameters of normal CSF.

Ans.

CSF	Normal
Pressure	50–250 mm of water
Color	Clear
White cell count (× 106/L)	0–4 all lymphocytes
Glucose	> 60% of blood level
Protein	< 0.45 gm/L
Microbiology	Sterile

Q.107. Tell the CSF findings in viral meningitis.

Ans.

Pressure	Normal
Appearance	Clear
Cells /μL	Upto 2000 lymphocytes
Protein(gm/L)	Normal
Glucose	Normal
Microbiology	Stain and culture—no organisms

Q.108. What are the common causes of bacterial meningitis?

Ans.

Age of onset	Common
i. Neonate	Gram-negative bacilli (*Escherichia coli, Proteus*) Group B streptococci
ii. Preschool child	*Haemophilus influenzae, Neisseria meningitidis, Streptococcus pneumoniae*
iii. Older child and adult	*Neisseria meningitidis, Streptococcus pneumoniae*

Q.109. If this patient develops maculopapular rash, what does it indicate?

Ans. Meningococcal septicemia and meningitis caused by *Neisseria meningitides.*

Q.110. What are the CSF findings in bacterial meningitis?

Ans.

Pressure	Usually increased/ normal
Appearance	Cloudy/turbid
Cells /μL	1000–5000 polymorphs
Protein(gm/L)	Increased
Glucose	Reduced
Microbiology	Gram stain +culture of organism

Q.111. Which antibiotic would you choose to treat pyogenic meningitis?

Ans.

Organism	Antibiotic
Unknown pyogenic	Cefotaxime
Meningococcus	Benzylpenicillin
Pneumococcus	Cefotaxime
Haemophilus	Cefotaxime

Q.112. Suppose you treat this patient, do you need any prophylaxis?

Ans. Yes.

Q.113. Which drugs are used in prophylaxis?

Ans. Oral rifampicin—Adult 600 mg 12-hourly for 2 days or a single dose of 500 mg of ciprofloxacin.

Q.114. What are the clinical features of tuberculous meningitis?

Ans. Symptoms—
- Headache
- Vomiting
- Low grade fever
- Depression of conscious level
- Confusion
- Behavior changes

Signs—
- Meningism (may be absent)
- Oculomotor palsies
- Papilledema
- Focal hemisphere sign.

Q.115. What are the CSF findings in tuberculous meningitis?

Ans.

Pressure	Usually increased/ normal
Appearance	Clear/ cloudy
Cells /µL	Upto 500 lymphocytes
Protein(gm/L)	Increased
Glucose	Reduced
Microbiology	Ziehl-Neelsen stain + culture

Q.116. What is cobweb?

Ans. There is formation of thin spidery web in the upper part of CSF of tuberculous meningitis if kept undisturbed in test tube.

Q.117. Difference between CSF of pyogenic and tubercular meningitis?

Ans.

Characteristics	Pyogenic meningitis	Tuberculous meningitis
Appearance	Cloudy/ turbid	Clear/ cloudy
Cells /µL	1000–5000 polymorphs	Upto 500 lymphocytes

Contd...

Contd...

Characteristics	Pyogenic meningitis	Tuberculous meningitis
Glucose	Markedly reduced	Reduced
Microbiology	Gram stain +culture of organism	Ziehl-Neelsen stain + culture— AFB

Q.118. How will you treat tuberculous meningitis?

Ans. Treat tubercular meningitis by giving category I for 9 months (2+7).

Q.119. What are the triad of Parkinson's disease?

Ans. Triad are:
- Bradykinesia.
- Resting tremor
- Rigidity.

Q.120. Which type of gait is in Parkinson's disease and describes the gait?

Ans. Festinant gait which is—
- Slow to start walking
- Shortened stride
- Rapid, small stride, tendency to shorten (festination)
- Reduced arm swinging
- Impaired balance on turning.

Q.121. Where is the lesion in Parkinson's disease?

Ans. Basal ganglia is the lesion Parkinson's disease.

Q.122. What is tremor? What are the causes of tremor?

Ans. Tremor is an oscillatory movement about a joint or a group of joints resulting from alternating contraction and relaxation of muscles.

Causes:
i. Resting tremor: Parkinson's disease.
ii. Tremor on out stressed hand: Anxiety, β-agonists (e.g. salbutamol), thyrotoxicosis, benign essential tremor.
iii. Intention tremor: Cerebellar disease.
iv. Flapping tremor/ asterixis:
   - Renal failure
   - Liver failure
   - Hypercapnia.

Q.123. Describe the tremor of Parkinson's disease.

Ans. Tremor of Parkinson's disease are:

- Coarse, complex movements, usually first in fingers/ thumb
- Flexion/extension of fingers
- Abduction/adduction of thumb
- Supination/pronation of forearm, producing in combination 'pill rolling movement'.

Q.124. How can you differentiate between thyrotoxic and Parkinson's tremor?

Ans.

Thyrotoxic tremor	Parkinson's tremor
Action tremor	Rest tremor
Usually symmetrical and bilateral	Asymmetrical and initially unilateral
Fine tremor(8–12 Hz)	Coarse tremor(4–6 Hz)
Diminished at rest	Diminished on action

Q.125. Which types of rigidity develop in Parkinson's disease?

Ans. Types are:

- Cogwheel type, mostly in upper limbs
- Plastic (lead pipe) type, mostly in legs.

Q.126. What are the investigations done in Parkinson's disease?

Ans. The diagnosis is made clinically, as there is no diagnostic test for Parkinson's disease.

Q.127. What are the drugs used in Parkinson's disease?

Ans. Drug therapy

i. Levodopa combined carbidopa.

ii. Anticholinergic drugs:
   - Trihexyphenidyl.
   - Orphenadrine.

iii. Amantidine.

iv. MAO—B inhibitors—Selegeline.

v. COMT inhibitors (Catechol-o-methyl transferase inhibitors).
   - Entacapone.

vi. Dopamine receptor agonists:
   - Bromocriptine
   - Pergolide
   - Cabergoline.

Q.128. What is asterixis? What are the causes?

Ans. On attempt to hold up the arms out with hands extended at the wrists, the posture is periodically dropped, allowing the hands to drop transiently before the posture is taken up again.

Causes are—
- Renal failure
- Liver failure
- Hypercapnia
- Drug toxicity, e.g. phenytoin
- Acute focal parietal or thalamic lesions.

Q.129. What is motor neuron disease (MND)?

Ans. Motor neuron disease is a progressive disorder of unknown cause, in which there is degeneration of motor neurons in the spinal cord and cranial nerve nuclei, and of pyramidal neurons in the motor cortex.

Q.130. What are the patterns of involvement in motor neuron disease?

Ans. Patterns of involment are:
i. Progressive muscular atrophy
ii. Progressive bulbar and pseudobulbar
iii. Amyotrophic lateral sclerosis
iv. Primary lateral sclerosis.

Q.131. What are the signs of cerebellar lesion?

Ans. Signs are:
- Titubation
- Nystagmus (horizontal)
- Scanning speech
- Intention tremor
- In co-ordination
- Dysdiadochokinesia
- Pastpointing
- Ataxia
- Hypotonia
- Pendular knee jerk.

CHAPTER 11

Skin

Q.1. Name some common skin problems.

Ans. Some common skin problems are:

- Scabies
- Eczema
- Psoriasis
- Taeniasis
- Urticaria/angioedema
- Pityriasis versicolor
- Lichen planus.

Q.2. A 10-year-old boy presents with itchy papules in finger webs, hands, also in the body, itching more intense at night. On examination, papules, vesicles, and pustules are present. What is your diagnosis?

Ans. Infected scabies is the diagnosis.

Q.3. What is the organism?

Ans. Organism is *Sarcoptes scabiei* homini.

Q.4. What is the diagnostic sign of scabies?

Ans. The pathognomonic sign is of linear or curved skin burrows.

Q.5. What are common sites for scabies?

Ans. Common sites are:

i. Webs of the fingers and toes
ii. On the palms and soles
iii. Around the wrists and axillae
iv. On the male genitalia
v. Around the nipples and umbilicus.

Q.6. How can you diagnose scabies?

Ans. Diagnosis is clinical (burrow and mite can be seen with hand lens).

Q.7. What are the complications of scabies?

Ans. Complications are:

- Secondary infection
- Glomerulonephritis (poststreptococcal).

Q.8. What type of complication is poststreptococcal glomerulonephritis ?

Ans. Poststreptococcal glomerulonephritis is an immune mechanism, not direct infection.

Q.9. How can you treat this case?

Ans. Treat by—

- 5% permethrin—Single application from neck to sole, may be repeated after a week.
- Phenoxymethyl penicillin—250 mg orally 6 hourly for 7 days to control infection.

Q.10. What are the other drugs used previously?

Ans. Other drugs are 25% benzyl benzoate, and monosulfirum.

Q.11. Describe a typical psoriatic lesion.

Ans. It is a well-demarcated erythematous patch with adherent silvery white scales.

Q.12. What are the types of psoriasis?

Ans. Types are:

- Stable plaque psoriasis
- Guttate psoriasis
- Erythrodermic psoriasis
- Pustular psoriasis.

Q.13. What are the common sites involved in psoriasis?

Ans. Scalp, elbows, knees, and lower back are the common sites involved in psoriasis.

Q.14. What are other organs involved in psoriasis?

Ans. Nails, joints, and eyes are other organs involved in psoriasis.

Q.15. What are the factors causing exacerbations of psoriasis?

Ans. Factors causing excerbations of psoriasis are:

- Trauma
- Infection
- Sunlight
- Drugs—Antimalarials, β-blockers, ACE inhibitors and lithium
- Emotion and anxiety.

Q.16. How can you treat psoriasis?

Ans. Treatment of psoriasis—

i. General measures:
- Explanation, reassurance, and instruction are vital.

ii. Specific measures:
- Topical and systemic.

Treatment categories in psoriasis—

i. Topical agents:
- Emollients, corticosteroids, vitamin D agonists, 'weak' tar or dithranol preparations.

ii. UV therapies:
- UVB or PUVA.

iii. Systemic agents:
- Methotrexate and retinoids
- Immunosuppressives, e.g. cyclosporine and mycophenolate
- Newer 'biological' agents, e.g. infliximab and etanercept.

iv. Intensive inpatient or day-patient care
Topical agents and UVR under medical supervision.

Q.17. What are the common sites of atopic eczema in children?

Ans. Backs of the knees, fronts of the elbows, wrists, and ankles are the common sites of atopic eczema in children.

Q.18. How can you differentiate eczema from ringworm clinically?

Ans.

Ringworm	Eczema
Well-demarcated raised margin	Ill-defined margin
Central healing	No central healing

Q.19. What is the organism responsible for ringworm?

Ans. Fungi, known as dermatophytes (microsporum, trichophyton, and epidermophyton).

Q.20. What are common sites for ringworm? Please tell the name according to their site.

Ans. Name of common sites according to their sites:

i. Surface of the body—Tinea corporis
ii. Groin—Tinea cruris
iii. Toe clefts—Tinea pedis
iv. Hands—Tinea manuum
v. Scalp—Tinea capitis.

Q.21. How can you treat ringworm?

Ans. Treatment can be given with—

i. Topical antifungal with terbinafine or miconazole cream with or without.
ii. Systemic with terbinafine, griseofulvin or itraconazole.

Q.22. Name some common bullous disease.

Ans. Common bullous diseases are:

- Bullous pemphigoid
- Pemphigus
- Dermatitis herpetiformis
- Epidermolysis bullosa acquisita.

Q.23. What are the common clinical presentation of chronic arsenicosis?

Ans. i. Melanosis—Hyperpigmentation interspersed with hypopigmented area giving rise to 'rain drop' pigmentation.
ii. Hyperkeratosis of palm and sole.

Q.24. Please name some sexually transmitted infections (STI).

Ans. **Bacterial**

Gonorrhea (*Neisseria gonorrhoeae*)
Syphilis (*Treponema pallidum*)
Chancroid (*Haemophilus ducreyi*)
Chlamydia (*Chlamydia trachomatis*)
Granuloma inguinale (*Klebsiella granulomatis*).

Fungal

Candidiasis (yeast infection).

Viral

Viral hepatitis (hepatitis B virus)
Herpes simplex (herpes simplex virus 1, 2)
HIV (human immunodeficiency virus)
HPV (human papilloma virus)
Molluscum contagiosum virus (MCV).

Parasites

Crab louse or 'pubic lice' (phthirus pubis)
Scabies (*Sarcoptes scabiei*).

Protozoal

Trichomoniasis (*Trichomonas vaginalis*).

Q.25. What is the difference between veneral disease and sexually transmitted disease (STD)?

Ans. No difference, two different terms for same problems.

Until the 1990s, STDs were commonly known as venereal diseases, then STD was used and in recent years the term sexually transmitted infections (STIs) has been preferred, as it has a broader range of meaning; sometimes the terms sexually transmitted infections (STI) and sexually transmitted diseases (STD) are used interchangeably.

Sexually transmitted infection is a broader term than sexually transmitted disease. An infection is colonization by a parasitic species, which may not cause any adverse effects. In a disease, the infection leads to impaired or abnormal function.

Q.26. How will you diagnose a case of gonorrhea?

Ans. Diagnosis of gonorrhea—

i. History of sexual exposure.
ii. Typical clinical presentation—Mucopurulent or purulent urethral discharge in male.
iii. Detection of gram-negative intracellular diplococci by microscopy of Gram stained prostatic smear or vaginal swab.

Q.27. Which organism is responsible for gonorrhea?

Ans. *Neisseria gonorrhoeae*—A gram-negative diplococci.

Q.28. Which specimen will you collect from the patient for diagnosis of gonorrhea?

Ans. Specimens are:

i. Prostatic smear or vaginal swab

ii. Urethral discharge
iii. Pharyngeal smear.

Q.29. What are the investigations to confirm the diagnosis?

Ans. Investigations are:

i. GNDC (gram-negative diplococci) on microscopy of smears from infected sites.
ii. Culture.
iii. NAAT (nucleic acid amplification test such as PCR).

Q.30. How can you treat gonococcal urethritis?

Ans. Treatments are:

i. Uncomplicated infection:
  - Cefixime 400 mg stat or
  - Ciprofloxacin 500 mg orally stat or
  - Ofloxacin 400 mg orally stat.

ii. If quinolone resistance:
  - Ceftriaxone 250 mg IM stat or
  - Spectinomycin 2 g IM stat.

Q.31. When is doxycycline used in gonococcal urethritis?

Ans. Doxycycline is used for treatment of chlamydia in gonococcal urethritis because concurrent infection is present in upto 50% of men with gonorrhea. Nongonococcal, nonchlamydial urethritis is also treated as for chlamydia.

Q.32. What is ophthalmia neonatorum?

Ans. Gonococcal ophthalmia neonatorum is gonococcal conjunctivitis of newborn contacting infection from mother following vaginal delivery and presents with purulent conjunctivitis and edema of the eyelids.

Q.33. What is classification of syphilis?

Ans. Classification of syphilis—

Stage	Acquired	Congenital
Early	Primary Secondary Latent	Clinical and latent
Late	Latent Benign tertiary Cardiovascular Neurosyphilis	Clinical and latent

Q.34. What is the organism of syphilis?

Ans. *Treponema pallidum* is the organism of syphilis.

Q.35. Which type of organism is it?

Ans. Spirochete.

Q.36. What is primary chancre?

Ans. The primary chancre is an indurated ulcer (primary lesion) which develops at the site of infection, usually in the genital area.

Q.37. How will you differentiate primary chancre from chancroid?

Ans.

Character	Primary chancre	Chancroid
Ulcer	A single painless indurated ulcer	Single or multiple painful ulcers with ragged undermined edges
Lymph node	Painless, nontender, mobile, discrete and rubbery	Tender, usually unilateral, unilocular, suppurative

Q.38. What is the drug of choice in the treatment of syphilis?

Ans. Penicillin is the drug of choice in the treatment of syphilis.

CHAPTER 12

Infectious Diseases

Q.1. Which infectious diseases have you seen in the medicine ward?

Ans. Enteric fever, malaria, kala-azar, and tuberculosis are the infectious diseases.

Q.2. What is enteric fever?

Ans. Fever caused by infection with *Salmonella typhi,* and *S. paratyphi* A and B is called enteric fever.

Q.3. What are the types?

Ans. Types are:
Typhoid fever —Caused by *Salmonella typhi*
Paratyphoid fever—Caused by *Salmonella paratyphi* A and B.

Q.4. What is the mode of transmission?

Ans. Feco-oral route.

Q.5. Tell some infections transmitted by feco-oral route.

Ans. Salmonella infection, bacillary dysentery (shigella), amebic dysentery, cholera, giardiasis, hepatitis A,E are the infections transmitted by feco-oral route.

Q.6. What is incubation period?

Ans. Incubation period is the period between the invasion of tissue by pathogen and the appearance of clinical features of infection.

Q.7. What is the incubation period of typhoid fever?

Ans. 10–14 days is the incubation period of typhoid fever.

Q.8. What are the clinical features of 1st week of typhoid fever?

Ans. Clinical features are:

- Fever
- Headache
- Myalgia
- Relative bradycardia
- Constipation
- Diarrhea and vomiting in children.

Q.9. What are the clinical features of end of 1st week of typhoid fever?

Ans. Clinical features are:
- Rose spots on trunk
- Splenomegaly
- Cough
- Abdominal distension
- Diarrhea.

Q.10. Which type of fever occurs in typhoid fever?

Ans. Continued type of fever occurs in typhoid fever.

Q.11. What is relative bradycardia?

Ans. When pulse rate does not increase to the expected level in comparison to rise of temperature. Pulse increases 10 beats/min for 1°C rise of temperature.

Q.12. What are the bowel complications of typhoid fever?

Ans. Bowel complications are—
- Perforation
- Hemorrhage.

Q.13. What are the systemic complications of typhoid fever?

Ans. Systemic complications are:
- Bone and joint infection—Osteomyelitis and septic arthritis
- Meningitis
- Cholecystitis
- Myocarditis
- Nephritis
- Chronic carriage.

Q.14. What are the investigations done in typhoid fever?

Ans. Investigations are:

1st week—
- Blood culture
- CBC.

2nd week—
- Stool culture
- Blood culture
- Urine culture
- Widal test.

Q.15. What are the antigens in Widal test?

Ans. Antigens are:
- Somatic antigen—O
- Flagellar antigen—H.

Q.16. What are the interpretations of Widal test?

Ans. Interpretations:

i. Four fold rise or rising titer is significant.

ii. High TO titer (e.g. 1:160 or more) indicates salmonella infection.

iii. High TO titer (e.g. 1:160 or more) and high TH titer(e.g.1:160) signifies *Salmonella typhi* infection.

iv. High TO titer (e.g. 1:160 or more) but low TH titer (e.g. <1:160) means salmonella infection but other than typhi.

v. Low TO titer (e.g. <1:160) but high TH titer (e.g. 1:160 or more) indicates anamnestic reaction, i.e. due to antigenic similarity.

Q.17. What is the definitive diagnosis?

Ans. Blood culture.

Q.18. What is the finding in CBC?

Ans. Leukopenia with relative lymphocytosis.

Q.19. How can you treat enteric fever?

Ans. Treatments are:

Tab. ciprofloxacin 500 mg 12 hourly for 14 days (drug of choice).

In case of resistance
- Tab azithromycin 500 mg daily for 14 days or 1 gm daily for 5 days is used.
- Ceftriaxone or cefotaxime.

In chronic carrier state
- Ciprofloxacin for 4 weeks.
- Sometimes, cholecystectomy may be necessary.

Q.20. Define fever?

Ans. It may be defined as rise of temperature above normal, measured under standard condition due to elevated set point of thermoregulatory center of the hypothalamus.

Or

'Fever' implies an elevated core body temperature > 38.0°C, i.e. above the normal daily variation.

Q.21. What is the normal daily variation of body temperature?

Ans. The normal 'set-point' of core temperature is tightly regulated within 37 ± 0.5°C.

Q.22. What are the types of fever?

Ans. Types of fever are:

- Classical fever—Having regular pattern
- Unclassified fever—Having no regular pattern.

Q.23. What are the types of classical fever?

Ans. Types of classical fever are:

i. Continued fever—Temperature fluctuation is less than 1°C in 24 hours, e.g. typhoid fever, typhus fever.

ii. Intermittent fever—Fever persists for a few hours in a day. Temperature falls to normal each day.

   a. Quotidian fever—Fever comes daily, may be several times, e.g. liver abscess.

   b. Tertian fever—Fever comes every alternate day, i.e. 3 days pattern (fever-normal-fever), e.g. *P. vivax*, and *P. ovale* malaria.

   c. Quartan fever—4 days pattern (2 days fever-2 days normal, fever-normal-normal-fever), e.g. *P. malariae* malaria.

iii. Remittent fever—Daily fluctuation greater than 2°C but does not return to normal, e.g. pneumonia, and infective endocarditis.

Q.24. What is PUO?

Ans. A temperature above 38°C for more than 3 weeks, without diagnosis despite initial investigation during 3 days of inpatient care or after more than 2 outpatient visits.

Q.25. What are the causes of PUO?

Ans. Causes are:

i. Infections: Abscess(liver),TB, infective endocarditis, malaria, dengue, kala-azar, E.fever, HIV, UTI, arthritis, and osteomyelitis.
ii. Malignancy: Lymphoma, leukemia, hepatoma, and renal cell carcinoma.
iii. Connective tissue disorder: SLE, temporal arteritis, Rh.fever, and PAN.
iv. Miscellaneous.
v. Idiopathic.

Q.26. What are the common causes of fever with hepatosplenomegaly?

Ans. Common causes are:
- Kala-azar
- Malaria
- Lymphoma
- Leukemia.

Q.27. What are the common causes of fever with chills and rigors?

Ans. Common causes are:
- Acute pyelonephritis
- Malaria
- Deep abscess
- Cholangitis
- Viral fever.

Q.28. What is kala-azar?

Ans. Kala-azar is the visceral leishmaniasis caused by *Leishmania donovani.*

Q.29. What is the vector of kala-azar?

Ans. Female phlebotomine sandfly is the vector of kala-azar.

Q.30. What are the forms of Leishmania donovani?

Ans. The forms of Leishmania donovani are:
i. Promastigote—Flagellar promastigotes in female sandfly.
ii. Amastigote (LD body)—Aflagellar amastigotes in macrophages of human body.

Q.31. Which form is LD body?

Ans. Amastigote.

Q.32. What is the clinical presentation of kala-azar?

Ans. Clinical presentations are:

i. Fever—Initially high fever, usually accompanied by rigor and chills. Fever intensity decreases over time and patients may become afebrile for intervening periods ranging from weeks to months. This is followed by a relapse of fever.
ii. Weight loss despite good appetite.
iii. Anemia and bleeding.
iv. Massive splenomegaly and moderate hepatomegaly.

Q.33. What are the investigations done in kala-azar?

Ans. Investigations are:

i. Blood
   - WBC—Leukopenia with relative lymphocytosis and monocytosis
   - Hb% reduced
   - Platelet—Thrombocytopenia.
ii. Serodiagnosis—
   - ELISA
   - Immunofluorescence antibody test
   - Direct agglutination test (DAT)
   - Rapid immunochromatographic strip test (RK39).
iii. Demonstration of amastigotes (Leishman-Donovan bodies) in splenic smears, bone marrow or lymph node smears.
iv. Culture in NNN media.
v. PCR.

Q.34. What is DAT?

Ans. DAT means direct agglutination test; it is called direct as it uses promastigote as antigen.

Q.35. In field level, which investigation is used?

Ans. RK39.

Q.36. What are the complications of kala-azar?

Ans. Complications are:

- Secondary infections: TB, pneumonia, and dysentery
- Bleeding manifestation
- Anemia
- PKDL.

Q.37. Why does anemia occur in kala-azar?

Ans. It is due to

i. Hypersplenism
ii. Short lifespan of RBC
iii. Hemolysis
iv. Ineffective erythropoiesis.

Q.38. What is the treatment of kala-azar?

Ans. Treatment A-I: (1st line of treatment for kala-azar patients) oral miltefosine—100 mg daily for 28 days.
Treatment A-II: Sodium antimony gluconate (SAG) (100 mg/ml) 20 mg/kg body weight IM /IV for 28 days.
Treatment B: (2nd line of treatment) amphotericine-B.

Q.39. What is the contraindication of miltefosine?

Ans. Pregnancy.

Q.40. What are the side effects of sodium stibogluconate?

Ans. Side effects are:

- Arthralgias
- Myalgias
- Raised hepatic transaminases
- Pancreatitis
- ECG changes (T-wave inversion and reduced amplitude)
- Cardiotoxicity.

Q.41. How to assess the response of treatment?

Ans. Rule of 6

Within:

- 6 days: Fever subside and patient feels well-being.
- 6 weeks: No anemia, weight gain and spleen size decrease.
- 6 months: Absence of LD bodies in spleen and bone marrow.

Q.42. What is PKDL?

Ans. PKDL is the cutaneous lesion which develops after successful treatment of visceral leishmaniasis.

Q.43. What is the treatment of PKDL?

Ans. Treatment of PKDL is Inj. sodium stibogluconate 20 mg/kg body weight daily for 20 days, which should be repeated after 10 days interval. 6 cycles are usually given.

Q.44. What is the causative organism of malaria?

Ans. A protozoon parasite plasmodium.

Q.45. What are the species of plasmodium?

Ans. Species of plasmodium are:

i. *P. falciparum*
ii. *P. vivax*
iii. *P. ovale*
iv. *P. malariae.*

Q.46. What is the vector of malaria?

Ans. Female anopheline mosquito is the vector of malaria.

Q.47. What types of malaria are common in Bangladesh?

Ans. Types are:

- *Plasmodium vivax* malaria
- *Plasmodium falciparum* malaria.

Q.48. Which type of fever occurs in falciparum malaria?

Ans. Irregular fever—Fever has no definite pattern in falciparum malaria.

Q.49. Which type of fever occurs in vivax malaria?

Ans. Tertian fever occurs in vivax malaria.

Q.50. What is cerebral malaria?

Ans. Any alteration of neurological status in a patient having *P. falciparum* is cerebral malaria.

Cerebral malaria is manifested by—

- Confusion
- Seizures
- Coma
- Usually no localizing signs.

Q.51. What are the causes of anemia in malaria?

Ans. Causes of anemia in malaria are:

i. Hemolysis of infected red cells
ii. Hemolysis of noninfected red cells (black water fever)
iii. Dyserythropoiesis
iv. Splenomegaly and sequestration
v. Folate depletion.

Q.52. What do you mean by relapse and recrudescence?

Ans. **Relapse**: It is the repeated attack of malaria due to persistence of exoerythrocytic forms in the liver as hypnozoites, causing reappearance of parasites in blood months or years later during which there was no parasitemia in blood. It occurs in *Plasmodium vivax* and *Plasmodium ovale.*

Recrudescence: It is the clinical manifestation results from multiplication of parasites in red cells which have not been eliminated by treatment and immune process. It is found in *P. falciparum* and *P. malariae.*

Q.53. What investigations are done to diagnose malaria?

Ans. Investigations are:
- Thick and thin blood films
- Immunochromatographic tests for malaria antigens.

Q.54. Why thick and thin film are done in malaria?

Ans. Thick and thin film are done in malaria because of—
- i. In thick film, erythrocytes are lysed releasing all blood stages of parasite, it is helpful to detect the parasite, even with low level of parasitemia.
- ii. Thin film is necessary to detect the species and also to quantify the parasite load in *Plasmodium falciparum.*

Q.55. How can you treat *P. vivax* malaria?

Ans. Chloroquinine 3 days + primaquine (radical cure) 14 days.

Chloroquinine—

Dose schedule:

1st day:	4 tabs
2nd day:	4 tabs
3rd day:	2 tabs
Primaquine—	15 mg daily for 14 days.

Q.56. What is radical cure?

Ans. It means eradication of malarial parasite called hypnozoite from the liver. It is treated with primaquine 15 mg daily for 14 days.

Q.57. How can you treat uncomplicated falciparum malaria?

Ans. 1st line treatment:

Artemether + lumefantrine combination (coartem)

Dose: 6 divided doses over 3 days

If for any reason coartem cannot be given then

2nd line treatment:

Quinine—10 mg/kg 8 hourly for 7 days (Q7).

If failure occurs after use of both quinine and coartem schedule or if after using quinine for 7 days and coartem cannot be used for any reason, then Q7+T7 or Q7+D7 7 days of oral quinine will be followed by 7 days of Tetracycline or doxycycline in case of 2nd line treatment failure 7 days of oral quinine and 7 days of tetracycline will be given simultaneously in case of 1st line treatment failure.

Q.58. How can you treat cerebral malaria?

Ans. Treatment of cerebral malaria—

i. By intravenous artesunate
   Or
   Quinine salt—10 mg/kg IV 8 hourly till patient can swallow, then orally.

ii. Supportive measures.

Q.59. How can you give quinine in cerebral malaria?

Ans. Treatment is started with a loading dose of 20 mg/kg quinine salt in 500 ml of D/A and infusion is given over 4 hours, then maintenance dosage at 10 mg/kg quinine salt is repeated at intervals of 8–12 hours until the patient can take drugs orally.

Q.60. Why is quinine used in DA?

Ans. Quinine is given in dextrose aqua infusion because quinine may cause hypoglycemia.

Q.61. What are the complications of *P. falciparum*?

Ans. Complications are:

- Coma (cerebral malaria)—Most common
- Hyperpyrexia
- Convulsions
- Hypoglycemia
- Severe anemia
- Acute pulmonary edema
- Acute renal failure
- Spontaneous bleeding and coagulopathy
- Metabolic acidosis
- Shock (algid malaria)
- Aspiration pneumonia.

Q.62. What is the chemoprophylaxis of malaria?

Ans. Clinical attacks of malaria may be preventable with drugs which is known as chemoprophylaxis.

Q.63. Which drugs are used for chemoprophylaxis?

Ans. Drugs are:

- Proguanil
- Malarone
- Doxycycline
- Chloroquine
- Mefloquine.

Q.64. How long is chemoprophylaxis given?

Ans. Chemoprophylaxis is begun 1 week before entering the malarious area and is continued for 4 weeks after leaving it.

Q.65. A 30-year-old male presents with few hypopigmented patches. There is loss of sensation over patches. What is your diagnosis?

Ans. Leprosy is the diagnosis.

Q.66. Define leprosy?

Ans. Leprosy (Hansen's disease) is a chronic granulomatous disease caused by *Mycobacterium leprae.*

Q.67. Which organs are mainly involved by leprosy?

Ans. Organs are:

- Skin
- Nerves.

Q.68. Which nerves are commonly affected in leprosy?

Ans. Nerves are commonly affected in leprosy are:

- Ulnar nerve (elbow)
- Median nerve (wrist)
- Radial nerve (humerus)— Wrist drop
- Common peroneal (knee)
- Great auricular nerve (posterior triangle of neck).

Q.69. Classify leprosy?

Ans. Classifications of leprosy:

i. WHO classification:
   a. Paucibacillary leprosy: It has 2–5 lesions with no bacilli.
   b. Multibacillary leprosy: 6 or more lesions which may have bacilli.
   c. Paucibacillary single lesion leprosy.

ii. Ridley-Jopling classification / Classification according to disease spectrum:

a. Tuberculoid (TT) leprosy
b. Borderline tuberculoid(BT) leprosy
c. Borderline borderline (BB) leprosy
d. Borderline lepromatous (BL) leprosy
e. Lepromatous (LL) leprosy.

Q.70. What are the cardinal features of leprosy?

Ans. Cardinal features are:
Hypopigmented anesthetic patch in the skin
Thickend peripheral nerves and loss of nerve function
Acid-fast bacilli on skin smears or biopsy.

Q.71. How can you confirm your diagnosis?

Ans. Diagnosis can be confirmed by detecting acid and alcohol fast bacilli in slit skin smear.

Q.72. From where slit skin smear is taken?

Ans. Slit skin smear is taken from—
- Skin lesion
- Ear lobule
- Tip of the nose
- Dorsum of fingers.

Q.73. What are the differential diagnoses for leprosy?

Ans. Differential diagnoses are:
- Fungal infection
- Tinea versicolor
- Drug reaction
- Eczema.

Q.74. How can you treat leprosy?

Ans. According to WHO:

Types of leprosy	Monthly supervised drug treatment	Daily self-administered drug treatment	Duration of treatment
Paucibacillary(2–5 skin lesions)	Rifampicin 600 mg	Dapsone 100 mg	6 months
Multibacillary (>5 skin lesions)	Rifampicin 600mg Clofazimine 300 mg	Clofazimine 50 mg Dapsone 100 mg	12 months

Contd...

Contd...

Types of leprosy	Monthly supervised drug treatment	Daily self-administered drug treatment	Duration of treatment
Paucibacillary single-lesion leprosy (one skin lesion)	Ofloxacin 400 mg Rifampicin 600 mg Minocycline 100 mg		Single dose

Q.75. Define food poisoning? What are the infective causes of food poisoning?

Ans. Acute gastroenteritis caused by ingestion of food or drink contaminated with living bacteria or their toxins.
Organisms:
Rotavirus
Campylobacter
Salmonella
Verocytotoxigenic *E. coli*
Shigella
Clostridium difficile
V. cholerae.

Q.76. What is dysentery?

Ans. It means presence of mucus with/without blood in stool.

Q.77. What are the causes of dysentery?

Ans. Causes are:

- Bacillary dysentery—Shigella,
- Amebic dysentery: *E. hystolytica.*

Q.78. How can you differentiate clinically?

Ans.

Traits	Amebic dysentery	Bacillary dysentery
Number of motion	6–8/day	Over 10 times
Amount	Copious	Small
Odor	Offensive	Odorless
Color	Dark red	Bright red
Nature	Blood and mucus mixed with feces	Blood and mucus no feces
Tennismus	Absent	Present

Q.79. How can you treat bacillary dysentery?

Ans. Correction of dehydration by oral rehydration therapy or, intravenous fluid if severe.

Antibiotic therapy with ciprofloxacin (500 mg 12-hourly for 3 days).

Q.80. What are the common causes of fever with maculopapular rash?

Ans. Causes are:

- Dengue fever
- Meningococcal septicemia.

Q.81. What is the causative agent of dengue fever?

Ans. Dengue virus—A flavivirus.

Q.82. What is the vector of dengue virus?

Ans. Ades mosquito is the vector of dengue virus.

Q.83. What is the habit of biting?

Ans. They bite at dusk and dawn.

Q.84. What is dengue syndrome?

Ans. Dengue syndrome encompasses—

i. Dengue fever (DF)
ii. Dengue hemorrhagic fever (DHF)
iii. Dengue shock syndrome (DSS).

Q.85. What are the criteria of dengue fever?

Ans. Dengue fever is an acute febrile illness of 2–7 days duration sometimes with two peaks having the following manifestations:

1. Sudden onset continuous fever
2. Two or more of the following features:
   a. Severe headache
   b. Retro-orbital pain
   c. Severe myalgia/arthralgia/back pain
   d. Hemorrhagic manifestations
   e. Nausea/vomiting/abdominal pain
   f. Leukopenia.
3. High index of suspicion based on period, population and place.
4. Absence of convincing evidence of any other febrile illness.

Q.86. How can you treat dengue fever?

Ans. Treatments:

Symptomatic and supportive

- Rest
- Antipyretic therapy for fever above 39°C
- Sponging with tepid water at room temperature
- Paracetamol (not more than 4 times in 24 hours)
- No aspirin or any other NSAID
- No antibiotics as these do not help.

Q.87. What is the difference between infectious and contagious disease?

Ans. Infectious diseases are caused by micro-organism (such as bacteria or viruses) that get into the body and cause illness.

Infectious diseases that spread from person to person are called contagious diseases. All contagious diseases are infectious but not all infectious diseases are contagious.

Q.88. Please name some contagious diseases.

Ans. Flu, common cold, or strep, sore throat, and diphtheria are some contagious diseases.

Q.89. What are bacteremia and septicemia?

Ans. Bacteremia refers to a bacterial invasion into blood circulation. Septicemia is bacteremia with replicating bacteria to cause an infection.

Q.90. What is superinfection? Name few organisms causing superinfection.

Ans. Superinfection is a new infection occurring in a patient having a pre-existing infection, e.g. bacterial superinfection in viral respiratory disease or infection of a chronic hepatitis B carrier with hepatitis D virus.

Q.91. Please name some drugs causing immune suppression.

Ans. Name of drugs are:

- Glucocorticoids
- Cytotoxics—Cyclophosphamide
- Cyclosporine
- Methotrexate
- Tacrolimus
- Mycophenolate.

Q.92. What are the causes of fever with rashes?

Ans. Causes are:

i. Macular or maculopapular
   - Measles
   - Infectious mononucleosis
   - Typhoid and paratyphoid fevers
   - Rickettsial infections
   - Dengue fever.

ii. Hemorrhagic
   - Meningococcal infection
   - Leptospirosis.

iii. Vesicular/pustular
   - Chickenpox.

Q.93. Which type of virus is measles?

Ans. Measles is a type of RNA virus.

Q.94. What are the features of measles?

Ans. Features are:

The incubation period is 8–14 days.

i. Prodormal and catarrhal stage—Malaise, fever, rhinorrhea, cough, conjunctival congestion and Koplik's spots.

ii. Eruptive or exanthematous stage—Maculopapular rash that initially occurs on the face, chiefly the forehead, and then spreads rapidly to involve the rest of the body.

Q.95. What is Koplik's spot? Where is it found? When it will be found?

Ans. Koplik's spots are small, grayish, irregular lesions surrounded by an erythematous base and are found on the buccal mucous membrane opposite the second molar tooth.

They occur a day or two before the onset of the rash.

Q.96. What are the complications of measles?

Ans. Compilcations are:

- Bacterial pneumonia
- Bronchitis
- Otitis media
- Gastroenteritis
- Myocarditis

- Hepatitis
- Enccphalitis
- Encephalomyelitis
- Subacute sclerosing panencephalitis (SSP).

Q.97. Name some common helminths in Bangladesh.

Ans. Some common helminths in Bangladesh are:
Ancylostoma duodenale
Ascaris lumbricoides
Enterobius vermicularis
Trichuris trichiura.

CHAPTER 13

Poisoning

Q.1. Please tell the principles of management of poisoning.

Ans. i. Resuscitation if needed (ABC): Maintenance of
- Airway
- Breathing
- Circulation.

ii. Elimination of the poison
  a. Surface decontamination
  b. Mouth: By stomach wash or induction of vomiting Activated charcol
  c. Urine: Fluid + diuretics— Forced diuresis and urinary alkalinization.

iii. Use of specific antidotes
OPC poisoning: Atropine and pralidoxime.

iv. Symptomatic management
If convulsion—Anticonvulsant and maintenance of nutrition.

v. Rehabilitation
- Personal
- Familial
- Social
- Occupational.

Q.2. What are the features of OPC poisoning?

Ans. Features are:

i. Muscarinic (DUMBEL)
- Diarrhea
- Urination
- Miosis
- Bronchospasm

- Emesis
- Lacrimation
- Salivation
- Bradycardia

ii. Nicotinic
- Muscle twiching
- Cramp
- Fasciculation
- Weakness of respiratory muscle.

iii. CNS
- Confusion
- Slurring of speech
- Headache
- Convulsion
- Coma.

Q.3. How can you treat this patient?

Ans. Treatments—

i. Initial stabilization—
- Clear airway (check oropharyngeal secretion, bronchospasm, and respiratory muscle paralysis).
- Improve oxygenation (oxygen therapy).

ii. Reduction of exposure—
- Washing with soap and tepid water
- Lavage within 1–2 hours.

iii. Antidote
- 2 antidotes—
  - Atropine (competative antagonism of M receptor)– Reverse muscarinic effect.
  - Oxime (reactivate ACh)—Reverse nicotinic effect.

iv. Supportive—
- Maintain circulation: 500–1000 mL of N/S over 20 minutes initially.
- Maintain respiratory insufficiency: Artificial respiration.
- Treatment of convulsion: Diazepam—10–20 mg IV or per rectum.
- Fluid and electrolyte balance.
- Control of infection—Aspiration: Antibiotic.
- Maintain nutrition.

Q.4. How atropine and pralidoxime is given in OPC poisoning?

Ans. Atropine (1 ampule contains 0.6 mg)

Atropine: 0.6 – 2 mg IV, repeat every 10 – 25 minutes until signs of atropinization. It should be maintained upto 48 – 72 hours.

Specific antidote pralidoxime: 1.5–2 gm IV over 4 minutes, repeat 4–6 hours and should be given before aging.

Q.5. What are the signs of atropinization?

Ans. Signs are:

- Mydriasis
- Tachycardia
- Flashing
- Dry mouth and axillae
- Anhidrosis and bronchodilation.

Q.6. What are the causes of death in OPC poisoning?

Ans. Causes are:

Immediate:

- Convulsion
- Cardiac arrhythmia
- Respiratory arrest.

Late:

- Renal failure.

Q.7. What is the common poisoning in childhood?

Ans. Kerosine is the common poisoning in childhood.

Q.8. A 3-year-old boy ingests kerosine accidentally and is brought to you. Will you give stomach wash?

Ans. No.

Q.9. This patient is well and running and playing after 4 hours. What will you do?

Ans. Observation.

Q.10. What are the clinical features of kerosine poisoning?

Ans. Clinical features are:

- Vomiting
- Cough
- Choking
- Wheezing

- Dyspnea
- Chemical pneumonitis.

Q.11. How can you manage kerosine poisoning?

Ans. Management of kerosine poisoning—

- Oxygen inhalation
- Gastric lavage contraindicated
- Broad spectrum antibiotic
- Nebulized bronchodilators
- X-ray chest for follow-up.

Q.12. How will you manage a patient of stupefying poisoning?

Ans. i. Resuscitation if needed (ABC): Maintenance of—
   - Airway
   - Breathing
   - Circulation.

ii. Elimination of the poison—
   - Fluid + diuretics—Forced diuresis, urinary alkalinization.

iii. Symptomatic management—
   - Maintenance of nutrition, fluid, and electrolytes
   - Condom catheterization (in male).

Q.13. What is diazepam poisoning?

Ans. When a person intake an amount of diazepam intentionally or accidentally more than prescribed or usual dose. It is better to tell overdose.

Q.14. What is the lethal dose of diazepam?

Ans. A lethal dose of diazepam is between 720–1240 mg/kg.

Q.15. What are the clinical features of diazepam poisoning?

Ans. Clinical features are:

- Drowsiness, ataxia, and confusion.
- In severe poisoning in susceptible groups, respiratory depression, and hypotension may occur.

Q.16. How will you manage this patient?

Ans. Managements—

i. Supportive—
   a. Activated charcoal within 1 hour.

b. Conscious level and oxygen saturation should be monitored for at least 6 hours after substantial overdose.

ii. Specific—Benzodiazepines antagonist—flumazenil.

Q.17. A man is brought to emergency with history of snake bite 3 hours back. On examination, cyanosis, ptosis, dribbling of saliva are found and patient cannot hold his head upright. What do you think?

Ans. Poisonous snake bite.

Q.18. How can you manage?

Ans. Managements—

- Immobilization of bitten part
- Polyvalent antivenom
- Tetanus prophylaxis
- Antibiotic.

Q.19. What are the types of antivenom?

Ans. Types are:

i. Monovalent

ii. Polyvalent.

Q.20. How to differentiate poisonous and nonpoisonous snake bite clinically?

Ans. By features of envenomation—

Systemic features due to toxins:

i. Neurotoxin:
   - Ptosis (partial or complete)
   - Broken neck sign
   - Hematological abnormality:
     - Persistent bleeding from the site.

ii. Myotoxin:
   - Respiratory failure
   - Muscle necrosis (blackening of local site)
   - Dark color urine due to myoglobulinuria.

iii. Cardiotoxin:
   - Arrhythmia.

CHAPTER 14

Psychiatry

Q.1. Classify psychiatric disorder.

Ans. Classification of psychiatric disorders

Stress-related disorders

- Acute stress disorder
- Adjustment disorder
- Posttraumatic stress disorder.

Anxiety disorders

- Generalized anxiety
- Phobic anxiety
- Panic disorder
- Obsessive-compulsive disorder.

Affective (mood) disorders

- Depressive disorder
- Mania and bipolar disorder.

Schizophrenia and delusional disorders

Substance misuse disorders

- Alcohol
- Drugs.

Organic disorders

- Acute, e.g. delirium
- Chronic, e.g. dementia.

Disorders of adult personality and behavior

- Personality disorder
- Factitious disorder.

Eating disorders

- Anorexia nervosa
- Bulimia nervosa.

Somatoform disorders

- Somatization disorder
- Dissociative (conversion) disorder
- Pain disorder
- Hypochondriasis
- Body dysmorphic disorder
- Somatoform autonomic dysfunction.

Neurasthenia

Puerperal mental disorder.

Q.2. Define delusion, hallucination, and illusion.

Ans. Delusion—A delusion is a false belief.

Hallucination—Hallucinations are sensory perceptions which occur in the absence of external stimuli, e.g. hearing voices when no one is present.

Illusion—Illusions are abnormal perceptions of real stimuli.

Q.3. You saw mads in the street. What are the psychiatric reasons of madness?

Ans. Reasons are:

- Schizophrenia
- Acute mania.

Q.4. Two mads in the road, one is well-dressed and delivering lecture in road and other is dirty having no cloth. What are your diagnoses?

Ans. Diagnoses are:

- Well-dressed—Acute mania
- Dirty —Schizophrenia.

Q.5. What is schizophrenia?

Ans. Schizophrenia is a psychosis characterized by delusions, hallucinations, and lack of insight.

Q.6. Please tell the first-rank symptoms of acute schizophrenia.

Ans. A = Auditory hallucinations—second or third person.

B = Broadcasting, insertion/withdrawal of thoughts.

C = Controlled feelings, impulses or acts ('passivity' experiences/phenomena).

D = Delusional perception (a particular experience is bizarrely interpreted).

Q.7. What are the negative symptoms of chronic schizophrenia?

Ans. Negative symptoms are:

- Flattened (blunted) affect
- Apathy and loss of drive (avolition)
- Social isolation
- Poverty of speech
- Poor self-care.

Q.8. What is the treatment of schizophrenia?

Ans. Antipsychotic drugs is the treatment of schizophrenia.

Q.9. Please classify antipsychotic drugs according to groups.

Ans.

Groups	Drugs
Phenothiazine	Chlorpromazine
Butyrophenone	Haloperidol
Thioxanthenes	Flupenthixol decanoate
Diphenylbutylpiperidine	Pimozide
Substituted benzamides	Sulpiride
Dibenzodiazepines	Clozapine
Benzisoxazole	Risperidone
Thienobenzodiazepines	Olanzapine
Dibenzothiazepines	Quetiapine

Q.10. What are the second generation antipsychotic drugs?

Ans. Second generation antipsychotic drugs are:

- Clozapine
- Risperidone
- Olanzapine.

Q.11. What is the benefit of second generation antipsychotic over first generation?

Ans. Less extrapyramidal side effect is the benefit of second generation antipsychotic over first generation.

Q.12. Tell the common side effects of antipsychotic drugs.

Ans. Side effects are:

- Extrapyramidal effects
- Gynecomastia
- Galactorrhea

- Dry mouth
- Blurred vision
- Constipation
- Urinary retention.

Q.13. What are the extrapyramidal effects?

Ans. Extrapyramidal effects are:
- Parkinsonism
- Akathisia (motor restlessness)
- Acute dystonia
- Tardive dyskinesia
- Oculogyric crisis.

Q.14. A 13-year-old girl is brought to you with eyeballs rotate upward, patient cannot close eyes and face is grimacing. She gives history of taking metoclopramide for vomiting. What is your diagnosis?

Ans. Extrapyramidal side effect of metoclopramide is the diagnosis.

Q.15. How can you treat this patient?

Ans. Treated by—
- Reassurance
- Stop the drug
- Inj. procyclidine.

Q.16. How long should antipsychotic drugs be given?

Ans. To prevent relapse, this will usually be given for 1–2 years in a patient with first episode of schizophrenia, but in patients with multiple episodes, treatment may be required for many years.

Q.17. Classify psychotropic drugs.

Ans. Classifications—

Antipsychotic	Phenothiazines
	Butyrophenones
	Second-generation antipsychotics
Antidepressant	Tricyclics and related drugs
	Monoamine oxidase inhibitors
	Novel noradrenergic or serotonin re-uptake inhibitors
Mood-stabilizing	Lithium
	Carbamazepine

	Sodium valproate
	Lamotrigine
Antianxiety	Benzodiazepines
	β-adrenoceptor antagonists.

Q.18. Please tell the common types of anxiety disorder.

Ans. Common types of anxiety disorders are:

- Generalized anxiety disorder
- Phobic anxiety disorder
- Panic disorder.

Q.19. What are the features of generalized anxiety disorder?

Ans. Features are:

i. Psychological—
  - Apprehension
  - Irritability
  - Fear of impending disaster
  - Depersonalization.

ii. Somatic—
  - Palpitations
  - Tremor
  - Dizziness
  - Sweating
  - Frequent desire to pass urine
  - Chest pain
  - Initial insomnia
  - Breathlessness
  - Headache.

Q.20. Name two antianxiety drugs.

Ans. Two antianxiety drugs are:

- Benzodiazepines
- β-blocker such as propranolol.

Q.21. What are the differential diagnoses of generalized anxiety disorder?

Ans. Differential diagnoses are:

- Thyrotoxicosis
- Pheochromocytoma
- Alcohol withdrawal
- Paroxysmal atrial tachycardia.

Q.22. What are the mood or affective disorders?

Ans. Mood or affective disorders are:

- Unipolar depression
- Bipolar disorder
- Dysthymia.

Q.23. Please tell the clinical features of major depression.

Ans. To make a diagnosis of major depression, at least five of the following symptoms, including at least one of the first two, must be present nearly everyday over a 2 week period.

Diagnostic criteria—

i. Depressed mood most of the day.
ii. Markedly diminished interest in almost all activities of the day.
iii. Significant weight loss or weight gain (at least 5% in one month).
iv. Insomnia or hypersomnia.
v. Psychomotor retardation or agitation.
vi. Fatigue or loss of energy.
vii. Feelings of worthlessness or excessive guilt.
viii. Diminished ability to think or concentrate or indecisiveness.
ix. Recurrent thoughts of death or suicide; a suicide attempt or a specific plan for suicide.

Q.24. Please name antidepressant drugs.

Ans. Antidepressant drugs are:

- Tricyclics and related drugs—Amitryptylline
- Monoamine oxidase inhibitors
- Noradrenergic or serotonin re-uptake inhibitors—Sertraline.

Q.25. Please tell name of some mood-stablizing drugs.

Ans. Some mood-stabilizing drugs are:

- Lithium
- Carbamazepine
- Sodium valproate.

Q.26. What is somatoform disorder?

Ans. The essential feature of these disorders is somatic symptoms which are not explained by a medical condition and not better diagnosed as part of a depressive or anxiety disorder.

Q.27. What are the syndromes included within this category?

Ans. Syndromes are:

- Somatization disorder
- Dissociative (conversion) disorder
- Pain disorder
- Hypochondriasis
- Body dysmorphic disorder
- Somatoform autonomic dysfunction.

Q.28. What is dissociative (conversion) disorder or 'hysteria'?

Ans. It is characterized by a loss or distortion of neurological function not fully explained by organic disease.

Q.29. What are the common presentations of dissociative (conversion) disorder?

Ans. Common presentations are:

- Gait disturbance
- Loss of function in limbs
- Aphonia
- Nonepileptic seizures
- Sensory loss
- Blindness.

Q.30. What is obsessive compulsive disorder (OCD)?

Ans. An obsessional symptom is an unwanted thought or impulse which enters the subject's mind repeatedly in spite of his or her conscious resistance.

Compulsions are the retuals which are patterns of behavior developed to relieve the anxiety generated by the original obsession.

Q.31. What is the management of OCD?

Ans. i. Behavior therapy—It is the preferred treatment like graded exposure, response prevention, and modeling.

ii. Drugs—Clomipramine (anafranil)— 50–150 mg /day
Flavoxamine (relafin)—50–300 mg/day
Fluoxetine (prolert)— 20 mg/day.

Q.32. Please give an example of OCD?

Ans. Repeated hand washing after contact with something.

Q.33. Please tell some stress-related disorders.

Ans. Some stress-related disorders are:

- Acute stress disorder

- Adjustment disorder
- Posttraumatic stress disorder.

Q.34. What are puerperal mental disorders?

Ans. Puerperal mental disorders are:
- Postpartum blues
- Postpartum depression
- Puerperal psychosis.

CHAPTER 15

Obesity

Q.1. Define obesity.

Ans. Obesity is a medical condition in which excess body fat has accumulated to the extent that it may have an adverse effect on health, leading to reduced life expectancy and/or increased health problems.

Or

Overweight and obesity are defined as abnormal or excessive fat accumulation that presents a risk to health (WHO).

Q.2. What is body mass index (BMI)?

Ans. BMI = Weight in kilograms /height in meter^2.

Q.3. Please tell the BMI classifications.

Ans.

BMI	Classifications
< 18.5	Underweight
18.5–24.9	Normal weight
25.0–29.9	Overweight
30.0–34.9	Class I obesity
35.0–39.9	Class II obesity
≥ 40.0	Class III obesity

Q.4. What are the types of obesity depending on body fat distribution?

Ans. i. Central obesity—(abdominal, visceral, android or apple-shaped) obesity.

ii. Generalized obesity—Subcutaneous fat accumulation causing generalized (gynoid or pear-shaped) obesity.

Q.5. What are the endocrine causes of obesity?

Ans. Endocrine causes of obesity are:

- Hypothyroidism
- Cushing's syndrome
- Insulinoma.

Q.6. What are the drugs causing obesity?

Ans. Common drugs are—

- Tricyclic antidepressants
- Corticosteroids
- Sulfonylureas
- Sodium valproate
- Estrogen-containing contraceptive pill.

Q.7. What are the complications of obesity?

Ans. Complications are:

- Type 2 diabetes
- Coronary heart disease
- Hypertension
- Stroke
- Hyperlipidemia
- Liver fat accumulation
- Nonalcoholic steatohepatitis (NASH)
- Cirrhosis
- Exertional dyspnea
- Sleep apnea
- Respiratory failure (pickwickian syndrome)
- Mechanical effects of weight
- Urinary incontinence
- Osteoarthritis
- Varicose veins
- Hormone-dependent cancers (breast and uterus)
- Polycystic ovary syndrome (infertility and hirsutism)
- Psychological morbidity (low self-esteem and depression)
- Gallstones
- Colorectal cancer
- Skin infections (groin and submammary candidiasis, and hidradenitis).

CHAPTER 16

Genetics

Q.1. Please tell some genetic disorders.

Ans. Some genetic disorders are:
- Hemophilia
- Thalassemia
- Hereditary spherocytosis
- Neurofibromatosis
- Marfan's syndrome.

Q.2. Please name two autosomal dominant disorders.

Ans. Two autosomal dominant disorders are:
- Neurofibromatosis
- Marfan's syndrome.

Q.3. Please tell two autosomal recessive disorders.

Ans. Two autosomal recessive disorders are:
- Thalassemia
- Sickle cell anemia.

Q.4. Please name two X-linked recessive disorders.

Ans. Two X-linked recessive disorders are:
- Hemophilia
- Glucose-6-phosphate dehydrogenase deficiency.

Q.5. What are the characteristics of X-linked recessive disorder?

Ans. Characteristics are:

i. Females are carrier
ii. Males are sufferer
iii. Carrier females transmit the disease.

Q.6. What are the characteristics of autosomal recessive disorder?

Ans. Characteristics are:

i. Unaffected carrier individuals transmit disease.
ii. If both parents are carrier, then one-quarter of their offsprings are affected and one-half are carriers.
iii. Usually only one generation is affected.

Q.7. What are the characteristics of autosomal dominant disorder?

Ans. Characteristics are:

i. Consecutive generations affected
ii. Half of offsprings affected, male = female
iii. Unaffected individual cannot transmit the disease.

Q.8. Please tell genotype of normal male.

Ans. Genotype of normal male is 46XY.

Q.9. Please tell genotype of normal female.

Ans. Genotype of normal female is 46XX.

Q.10. Classify chromosomal disorder with example.

Ans. Classifications:

i. Numerical abnormalities—
   - Trisomy 21 (47, XY, +21)— Down's syndrome
   - 47, XXY— Klinefelter's syndrome
   - 45, X0— Turner's syndrome.

ii. Structural chromosomal aberrations
   - 46, XY, del (5p) Cri-du-chat syndrome, deletion of short arm of chromosome 5
   - 46, XY, t (9, 22) Philadelphia chromosome.

Q.11. What are the clinical features of Down's syndrome?

Ans. Clinical features of Down's syndrome are:

- Characteristic facies—Flat face, low set ear, epicanthic fold and widespaced eyes.
- Mental retardation.
- Single palmar crease (simian crease).
- Short stature.
- Fond of music.
- Congenital heart defects.

Q.12. What are the clinical features of Turner's syndrome?

Ans. Clinical features of Turner's syndrome are:

- Short stature
- Webbing of neck
- Cubitus valgus (increased carrying angle)
- Streak gonads
- Primary amenorrhea
- Aortic coarctation.

CHAPTER 17

Geriatric Problem

Q.1. What are the common geriatric problems?

Ans. Common geriatric problems are:

- Falls
- Urinary incontinence
- Arthritis
- Disability
- Hypertension
- Hearing impairment
- Heart disease
- Cataract
- Orthopedic impairment
- Depression
- Malignant neoplasm
- Diabetes mallitus
- Asthma and emphysema
- Alzheimer's disease
- Frailty
- Cardiovascular disease.

Q.2. What are the common causes of fall?

Ans. Common causes of fall are:

- Muscle weakness
- Gait or balance abnormality
- Visual impairment
- Arthritis
- Depression
- Cognitive impairment
- Drugs.

Q.3. Define postural hypotension?

Ans. Postural hypotension is defined as a drop in blood pressure of > 20 mm Hg systolic or > 10 mm Hg diastolic pressure on standing from supine.

Q.4. How can you manage postural hypotension?

Ans. Management—

i. Correction of dehydration.
ii. Head-up tilt of the bed.
iii. Support stockings (older patients may struggle to get these on).
iii. Nonsteroidal anti-inflammatory drugs (NSAIDs; increase circulating volume via salt and water retention; gastric and renal side effects limit use).
iv. Fludrocortisone (causes salt and water retention; often poorly tolerated due to fluid overload).
v. Midodrine (α-adrenergic agent).

CHAPTER 18

Immunity

Q.1. Define anaphylaxis.

Ans. Anaphylaxis is a potentially life-threatening, systemic allergic reaction caused by the release of histamine and other vasoactive mediators from mast cells.

Q.2. What are the common causes of anaphylaxis?

Ans. Common causes of anaphylaxis are:

- IgE-mediated mast cell degranulation
- Foods
- Peanuts
- Fish and shellfish
- Eggs
- Insect stings
- Bee venom
- Wasp venom
- Drugs
- Penicillin and aspirin and nonsteroidal anti-inflammatory drugs (NSAIDs).

Q.3. How can you manage?

Ans. Anaphylaxis is an acute medical emergency.

i. Prevent further contact with allergen, e.g. removal of bee sting.

ii. Ensure airway patency.

iii. Administer intramuscular adrenaline (epinephrine) promptly.

Adult dose: 0.3–1.0 mL 1:1000 solution, acts within minutes, repeat at 5–10 minutes intervals if initial response is inadequate.

iv. Administer antihistamines, e.g. chlorphenamine 10 mg IM or slow IV injection. Directly opposes effects of mast cell activation.

v. Administer corticosteroids, e.g. hydrocortisone 200 mg IV prevents rebound symptoms in severely affected patients.

vi. Provide supportive treatments, e.g. nebulized β_2-agonists to decrease bronchoconstriction.

vii. IV fluids to restore or maintain blood pressure.

viii. Oxygen.

Q.4. Please give one example for each hypersensitivity reaction.

Ans.

Types	Examples
I	Anaphylaxis
II	Blood transfusion reaction
III	Serum sickness
IV	Montoux test

CHAPTER 19

Environment

Q.1. What are the temperature-related disorders?

Ans. Temperature-related disorders are:

- Hypothermia
- Heat cramps
- Heat syncope
- Heat exhaustion
- Heat stroke.

Q.2. What is hypothermia?

Ans. When core temperature falls below 35°C, it is called hypothermia.

Q.3. What are the common causes of hypothermia?

Ans. Common causes are:

- Immersion in cold water
- Exposure to extreme climates such as during hill walking
- Hypothyroidism
- Glucocorticoid insufficiency
- Stroke
- Hepatic failure
- Hypoglycemia.

Q.4. What are the clinical features of hypothermia?

Ans. Clinical features are:

- Depressed conscious level
- Dehydration
- Confusion
- Muscle stiffness

- Ice cold and pale
- Bradycardia
- Hypotension.

Q.5. How can you treat hypothermia?

Ans. Treatments are:

i. Resuscitation-maintain ABC
ii. Rewarming the patient in a controlled manner
iii. Treatment of associated hypoxia (by oxygenation and ventilation if necessary), fluid and electrolyte disturbance and dysrhythmias if present.

Q.6. What are the heat-related illnesses?

Ans. Heat-related illnesses are:

- Heat cramps
- Heat syncope
- Heat exhaustion
- Heat stroke.

Q.7. What is heat stroke?

Ans. Heat stroke occurs when the core body temperature rises above 40°C and is a life-threatening condition.

Q.8. How can you treat heat stroke?

Ans. Treatments are:

i. The patient should be resuscitated with rapid cooling by spraying with water, fanning, and ice packs in the axillae and groins.
ii. Cold crystalloid intravenous fluids are given but solutions containing potassium should be avoided.

Q.9. What are the differences between heat stroke and heat exhaustion?

Ans. In heat stroke, core temperature is >40°C and sweating is absent but in heat exhaustion, core temperature is > 37–40°C and sweating is present.

Q.10. What is hyperthermia and hyperpyrexia?

Ans. Hyperthermia is an increase in body temperature over the body's thermoregulatory set-point, due to excessive heat production and/or insufficient thermoregulation. It is not a fever.

Hyperpyrexia is a fever with an extreme elevation of body temperature greater than or equal to 41.5°C (106.7°F).

Q.11. What is the difference between hyperthermia and hyperpyrexia?

Ans.

Hyperpyrexia	Hyperthermia
Hyperpyrexia is a fever	It is not a fever
Temperature is above the normal temperature but within thermoregulatory set-point	The body temperature rises above its set-point
Body generates heat to achieve this temperature	The body temperature rises due to an outside source

CHAPTER 20

Nutrition

Q.1. What are the fat-soluble vitamins?

Ans. Fat-soluble vitamins are vitamins A, D, E, and K.

Q.2. Please tell their deficiency diseases.

Ans.

Vitamins	Deficiency symptoms
Vitamin A	Night blindness Xerophthalmia Bitot's spots Keratomalacia Blindness
Vitamin D	Rickets and osteomalacia
Vitamin E	Mild hemolytic anemia, ataxia and visual scotomas
Vitamin K	Delayed coagulation and bleeding

Q.3. What are water-soluble vitamins?

Ans. Water-soluble vitamins are:

- Thiamin (vitamin B_1)
- Riboflavin (vitamin B_2)
- Niacin (vitamin B_3)
- Pyridoxine (vitamin B_6)
- Biotin
- Vitamin B_{12} and folate
- Vitamin C (ascorbic acid).

Q.4. What are the deficiency features of vitamin B_1 deficiency?

Ans. Deficiency features are:

Beriberi—

i. Dry (or neurological) beriberi—Chronic peripheral neuropathy and with wrist and/or foot drop. Korsakoff's psychosis Wernicke's encephalopathy.

ii. Wet (or cardiac) beriberi—Generalized edema due to biventricular heart failure with pulmonary congestion.

Q.5. What are the deficiency features of niacin deficiency?

Ans. Pellagra (the disease of the three Ds)— Dermatitis, diarrhea, and dementia.

Q.6. What are the deficiency features of vitamin C deficiency?

Ans. Scurvy is the deficiency features of vitamin C deficiency.

Q.7. What are the clinical features of scurvy?

Ans. Clinical features are—

i. Swollen gums which bleed easily
ii. Petechial and perifollicular hemorrhages giving rise to corkscrew hair
iii. Ecchymosis
iv. Hemarthrosis
v. Gastrointestinal bleeding
vi. Anemia
vii. Poor wound healing.

Q.8. What are the X-ray findings of scurvy?

Ans. X-findings are:

i. Epiphysis is ring-shaped, sclerotic and sharply demarcated(Wimberger's sign).
ii. Metaphysis is dense resembling a white line (white line of Frankle).
iii. Beneath metaphysic, a lucent zone(Trumerfeld zone) is present.
iv. There is spur at the corner(Pelkan's spur).

Q.9. How can you treat vitamin A deficiency?

Ans. Giving oral vitamin A supplement—100000 IU first day
100000 IU second day
100000 IU eighth day

Q.10. A boy ingests 20 vitamin A capsule. What may be the effects?

Ans. Acute overdose leads to nausea and headache, increased intracranial pressure and skin desquamation.

Q.11. A 30-year-old lady takes 4 capsules of vitamin A daily for long time due to misbelief of being beautiful. What may happen?

Ans. It can cause liver damage, hyperostosis, and teratogenicity.

Q.12. What are the deficiency features of vitamin D deficiency?

Ans. Deficiency features of vitamin D are:

- In children—Rickets
- In adult—Osteomalacia.

Q.13. Please tell the metabolism of vitamin D.

Ans. The main source of vitamin D in the body is synthesis of cholecalciferol from 7-dehydrocholesterol in the skin by the action of ultraviolet sunlight, a minor portion comes from diet. Cholecalciferol is inactive, which is converted first in the liver to 25-hydroxycholecalciferol ($25(OH)D_3$) and subsequently in the kidney (by the enzyme 1 hydroxylase) to 1,25-dihydroxycholecalciferol ($1,25(OH)2D_3$) which is active form of vitamin D.

Q.14. Please tell functions of vitamin D on intestine, bone and kidney.

Ans. Functions of vitamin D on—

Intestine—Vitamin D increases Ca^2+ absorption from the gut.

Bone—Vitamin D increases calcification of osteoid tissue and also bone resorption.

Kidney—Vitamin D increases calcium reabsorption and phosphate excretion.

Q.15. What are the X-ray findings of ricket?

Ans. X-ray findings are:

i. Widening, splaying, cupping, and irregularities of metaphysis.
ii. Distance between epiphysis and metaphysis is increased, i.e. zone of provisional calcification is lost.

Q.16. What are common nutritional disorders?

Ans. Common nutritional disorders are:

- Kwashiorkor

- Marasmus
- Iodine deficiency
- Night blindness due to vitamin A deficiency
- Iron deficiency anemia.

Q.17. What are the neurological deficits in nutritional deficiency?

Ans. Vitamin B_1 deficiency— Peripheral neuropathy
Korsakoff's psychosis
Wernicke's encephalopathy
Vitamin B_6 deficiency— Peripheral neuropathy
Niacin deficiency— Dementia
Vitamin B_{12} deficiency— Peripheral neuropathy
Subacute combined degeneration of spinal cord
Optic atrophy
Dementia.

Q.18. Which vitamin deficiency is more common either vitamin B_{12} or folic acid?

Ans. Folic acid deficiency is more common.

CHAPTER 21

Electrolytes

Q.1. What is the normal plasma sodium level?

Ans. Normal Na level: 135–145 mmol/L.

Q.2. What is hyponatremia?

Ans. When plasma sodium<135 mmol/L, then it is called hyponatremia.

Q.3. Classify hyponatremia

Ans. Classifications—

According to severity—

i. Mild hyponatremia: When sodium level is 130–135 mmol/L (S/S:Malaise, nausea).
ii. Moderate hyponatremia: When sodium level is 120–130 mmol/L (S/S: Headache, vomiting, lethargy).
iii. Severe hyponatremia: When sodium level is <120 mmol/L (S/S:Neurological manifestation like impaired consciousness, stupor, coma and seizure).
iv. Very severe hyponatremia: When Na level is <110 mmol/L.

Q.4. What are the features of severe hyponatremia (hyponatremic encephalopathy)?

Ans. Neurological dysfunction showing:

- Anorexia
- Nausea and vomiting
- Apathy
- Dizziness
- Confusion
- Convulsion
- Coma.

Q.5. How will you treat a case of hyponatremia?

Ans. Treatments arc:

i. If hyponatremia has developed rapidly (over hours to days), severe (<110 mmol/L) or presence of neurological features—Infusion of hypertonic (3%) sodium chloride solutions, the rate of correction of the plasma Na concentration should not exceed 0.5 mmol/L/hours.

ii. Treatment of underlying cause.

Q.6. What will be the result if correction of hyponatremia is done rapidly?

Ans. Rapid correction may lead to central pontine mylinolysis(osmotic demyelinating syndrome).

Q.7. What is iatrogenic hyponatremia?

Ans. Excess DA administration or sample collected from hand used for IV line.

Q.8. What is pseudohyponatremia?

Ans. Pseudohyponatremia is the spurious low value seen if a high proportion of the serum volume is free of water. For example severe hyperlipidemia.

Q.9. What is the normal plasma K level?

Ans. Normal plasma concentration 3.5–5 mmol/L.

Q.10. What is hyperkalemia?

Ans. When K+ level >5 mmol/L, then its called hyperkalemia.

Q.11. What are the types of hyperkalemia?

Ans. Types are:

- Mild hyperkalemia: 5–6 mmol/L
- Moderate hyperkalemia: 6–7 mmol/L
- Severe hyperkalemia: >7 mmol/L.

Q.12. What are the common causes of hyperkalemia?

Ans. Common causes are:

i. Renal impairment
  - Acute renal failure
  - Chronic renal failure

ii. Adrenocortical insufficiency (Addison's disease)

iii. Excess intake—
  - Exogenous—Dietary and IV therapy.
  - Endogenous—Hemolysis and rhabdomyolysis.

iv. Transcellular shift—Acidosis (diabetic ketoacidosis), insulin deficiency, hyperkalemic periodic paralysis.
v. Drugs—ACE inhibitor and potassium sparing diuretics.

Q.13. What are the ECG changes in hyperkalemia?

Ans. ECG changes are:
i. Tall peaked T-waves
ii. Wide QRS complexes
iii. Loss of P-wave
iv. Sine wave.

Q.14. How can you manage severe hyperkalemia?

Ans. Management—
Severe hyperkalemia—Urgent measures must be taken
i. Intravenous calcium gluconate (10 mL of 10% solution)—To stabilize conductive tissue membranes.
ii. Inhaled β_2 agonist, e.g. salbutamol.
or
Intravenous glucose (50 mL of 50% solution) and insulin (5 U Actrapid).
iii. Intravenous sodium bicarbonate (100 mL of 8.4% solution), if acidosis present.
iv. Remove K^+ from body, intravenous furosemide, and normal saline.
v. Ion-exchange resin (e.g. resonium) orally or rectally.
vi. Dialysis.

Q.15. What is spurious / pseudohyperkalemia?

Ans. During venepuncture for blood sample collection, due to incorrect/repeated handling there may be—
- Tissue damage
- RBC damage
- Endothelial cell damage
- Delayed processing.

This results in release of potassium and show hyperkalemia in blood sample, although patient's K^+ is normal.

Q.16. How will you treat a patient of hypokalemic?

Ans. Treatments are:
i. The underlying cause should be identified and treated if possible.

ii. Acute hypokalemia may correct spontaneously.
iii. In most cases, the oral administration of potassium supplements in the form of slow-release potassium or effervescent potassium, is sufficient.
iv. Intravenous potassium replacement is required only in conditions such as cardiac arrhythmias, muscle weakness or severe diabetic ketoacidosis.